Big Data in eHealthcare

Challenges and Perspectives

Big Data in eHealthcare
Challenges and Perspectives

Nandini Mukherjee
Sarmistha Neogy
Samiran Chattopadhyay

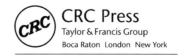

CRC Press
Taylor & Francis Group
Boca Raton London New York

CRC Press is an imprint of the
Taylor & Francis Group, an **informa** business

CRC Press
Taylor & Francis Group
6000 Broken Sound Parkway NW, Suite 300
Boca Raton, FL 33487-2742

© 2019 by Taylor & Francis Group, LLC
CRC Press is an imprint of Taylor & Francis Group, an Informa business

Printed on acid-free paper
Version Date: 20181122

International Standard Book Number-13: 978-0-8153-9440-2 (Hardback)

Library of Congress Cataloging-in-Publication Data

Names: Mukherjee, Nandini, author. | Neogy, Sarmistha, author. | Chattopadhyay, Samiran, author.
Title: Big data in eHealthcare : challenges and perspectives / Nandini Mukherjee, Sarmistha Neogy, Samiran Chattopadhyay.
Description: Boca Raton, FL : CRC Press/Taylor & Francis Group, 2019. | Includes bibliographical references and index.
Identifiers: LCCN 2019011925| ISBN 9780815394402 (hardback : acid-free paper) | ISBN 9781351057790 (ebook)
Subjects: LCSH: Medical informatics. | Medicine--Data processing. | Big data. | Data mining.
Classification: LCC R858 .M85 2019 | DDC 610.285--dc23
LC record available at https://lccn.loc.gov/2019011925

Visit the Taylor & Francis Web site at
http://www.taylorandfrancis.com

and the CRC Press Web site at
http://www.crcpress.com

To my daughter Shabnam and my husband Biman
— Nandini Mukherjee

To my daughter Roshni and my son-in-law Prince Bose
— Sarmistha Neogy

To my daughter Anwesha and my wife Matangini
— Samiran Chattopadhyay

Contents

List of Figures   xiii

Preface   xv

Acknowledgements   xvii

Authors   xix

1 Introduction   **1**

    1.1 What Is eHealth? 2
    1.2 eHealth Technologies 3
    1.3 eHealth Applications 4
       1.3.1 Health Informatics 5
       1.3.2 mHealth 5
       1.3.3 Telehealth 6
    1.4 eHealth and Big Data 8
    1.5 Issues and Challenges 9
    1.6 Chapter Notes 11

References   **12**

2 Electronic Health Records   **13**

    2.1 Introduction 13
    2.2 Electronic Health Records 14
    2.3 EHR Standards 16
       2.3.1 ISO 13606 17
       2.3.2 HL7 18
       2.3.3 OpenEHR 23
    2.4 Adoption of EHR Standards 30
    2.5 Ontology-based Approaches 32
       2.5.1 Developing an Ontology 33
       2.5.2 Ontologies for EHR 33
       2.5.3 Ontologies in Healthcare 34
    2.6 Chapter Notes 35

References   **40**

3   Big Data: From Hype to Action   **43**

   3.1   Introduction   43
   3.2   What Is Big Data?   44
   3.3   Big Data Properties   45
   3.4   Why Is Big Data Important?   47
   3.5   Big Data in the World   49
   3.6   Big Data in Healthcare   50
         3.6.1   Is Health Data Big Data?   51
         3.6.2   Big Data: Healthcare Providers   52
   3.7   Other Big Data Applications   54
         3.7.1   Banking and Securities   55
         3.7.2   Communications, Media, and Entertainment   55
         3.7.3   Manufacturing and Natural Resources   56
         3.7.4   Government   56
         3.7.5   Transportation   56
         3.7.6   Education   56
   3.8   Securing Big Data   57
         3.8.1   Security Considerations   57
         3.8.2   Security Requirements   58
         3.8.3   Some Observations   59
   3.9   Big Data Security Framework   59
   3.10 Chapter Notes   61

References   **62**

4   Acquisition of Big Health Data   **65**

   4.1   Introduction   65
   4.2   Wireless Body Area Network   66
         4.2.1   BAN Design Aspects   68
         4.2.2   WBAN Sensors   70
         4.2.3   Technologies for WBAN   70
                 4.2.3.1   Bluetooth and Bluetooth LE   70
                 4.2.3.2   ZigBee and WLAN   71
                 4.2.3.3   WBAN standard   71
         4.2.4   Network Layer   73
         4.2.5   Inter-WBAN Interference   74
   4.3   Crowdsourcing   76
   4.4   Social Network   79
   4.5   Chapter Notes   83

References   **84**

5   Health Data Analytics   87

5.1   Introduction   88
5.2   Artificial Neural Networks   90
    5.2.1   Model of an ANN   90
    5.2.2   Modes of ANN   92
    5.2.3   Structure of ANNs   93
    5.2.4   Training a Feedforward Neural Network   93
    5.2.5   ANN in Medical Domain   96
    5.2.6   Weakness of ANNs   97
5.3   Classification and Clustering   98
    5.3.1   Clustering via K-Means   99
    5.3.2   Some Additional Remarks about K-Means   100
5.4   Statistical Classifier: Bayesian and Naive Classification . . .   102
    5.4.1   Experiments with Medical Data   104
    5.4.2   Decision Trees   106
    5.4.3   Clasical Indction of Decision Trees   108
5.5   Association Rule Mining (ARM)   111
    5.5.1   Simple Approach for Rule Discovery   112
    5.5.2   Processing of Medical Data   113
    5.5.3   Association Rule Mining in Health Data   113
    5.5.4   Issues with Association Rule Mining   114
5.6   Time Series Analysis   115
    5.6.1   Time Series Regression Models   116
    5.6.2   Linear AR Time Series Models   117
    5.6.3   Application of Time Series   120
5.7   Text Mining   120
    5.7.1   Term Frequency and Inverse Document Frequency . .   122
    5.7.2   Topic Modeling   123
5.8   Chapter Notes   124

References   126

6   Architecture and Computational Models for Big Data Processing   129

6.1   Introduction   130
6.2   Performance Issues   130
6.3   Parallel Architecture   135
    6.3.1   Distributed Shared Memory   137
    6.3.2   Hierarchical Hybrid Architecture   138
    6.3.3   Cluster Computing   138
    6.3.4   Multicore Architecture   139
    6.3.5   GPU Computing   140
    6.3.6   Recent Advances in Computer Architecture   141

6.4   Exploiting Parallelism   142
6.5   MapReduce Overview   144
       6.5.1   MapReduce Programming Model   146
       6.5.2   MapReduce Framework Implementation   146
6.6   Hadoop   148
       6.6.1   Hadoop Architecture   149
       6.6.2   Resource Provisioning Framework   149
       6.6.3   Hadoop Distributed File System   151
       6.6.4   MapReduce Framework   152
       6.6.5   Hadoop Common   153
       6.6.6   Hadoop Performance   153
6.7   Hadoop Ecosystem   153
       6.7.1   Apache Spark   154
       6.7.2   Apache ZooKeeper   155
6.8   Streaming Data Processing   156
       6.8.1   Apache Flume   156
       6.8.2   Spark Streaming   158
       6.8.3   Amazon Kinesis Streaming Data Platform   159
6.9   Chapter Notes   159

References   **161**

7 Big Data Storage   **163**

7.1   Introduction   163
7.2   Structured vs. Unstructured Data   164
7.3   Problems with Relational Databases   165
7.4   NoSQL Databases   166
7.5   Document-oriented Databases   168
       7.5.1   MongoDB   169
       7.5.2   Apache CouchDB   173
7.6   Column-oriented Databases   174
       7.6.1   Apache Cassandra   174
       7.6.2   Apache HBase   179
7.7   Graph Databases   181
       7.7.1   Neo4j   181
7.8   Health Data Storage: A Case Study   184
7.9   Chapter Notes   188

References   **189**

8 Security and Privacy for Health Data   **191**

8.1   Introduction   192
       8.1.1   Security   192
       8.1.2   Privacy   193

8.1.3 Privacy-Preserving Data Management 194
8.1.4 A Few Common Questions 197
8.2 Security and Privacy Issues 198
8.2.1 Storage 199
8.2.2 Security Breach 199
8.2.3 Data Mingling 200
8.2.4 Data Sensitivity 200
8.2.5 User 202
8.2.6 Computations 202
8.2.7 Transaction Logs 202
8.2.8 Validation of Input 202
8.2.9 Data Mining 203
8.2.10 Access Control 203
8.2.11 Data Audit 204
8.2.12 Data Source 205
8.2.13 Security Best Practices 206
8.2.14 Software Security 207
8.2.15 Secure Hardware 207
8.2.16 User Account Management 207
8.2.17 Clustering and Auditing of Databases 208
8.3 Challenges 208
8.3.1 Malicious User 208
8.3.2 Identifying Threats 209
8.3.3 Risk Mitigation 209
8.3.4 Real-Time Monitoring 210
8.3.5 Privacy Preservation 210
8.3.5.1 Health Data Sale 212
8.3.5.2 Compliance for EHR 212
8.4 Security of NoSQL Databases 213
8.4.1 Reviewing Security in NoSQL databases 213
8.4.1.1 Security in Cassandra 214
8.4.1.2 Security in MongoDB 215
8.4.1.3 Security in HBase 216
8.4.2 Reviewing Enterprise Approaches towards Security in
NoSQL Databases 218
8.5 Integrating Security with Big Data Solutions 219
8.5.1 Big Data Enterprise Security 220
8.6 Secured Health Data Delivery: A Case Study 223
8.7 Chapter Notes 227

References **228**

Index **233**

List of Figures

1.1   eHealth sensors and medical IoT development platform . . .   4
1.2   Wearable technology   4
1.3   Issues in eHealth data   10

2.1   HL7 and OSI layers [Source: [18]]   19
2.2   Core classes of RIM   21
2.3   Entity class and its subclasses [Source: [28]]   22
2.4   Role class [Source: [28]]   23
2.5   Participation class and its subclasses [Source: [28]]   24
2.6   openEHR - multilevel modeling   25
2.7   OpenEHR reference model classes   27
2.8   OpenEHR reference model classes — an example   28
2.9   Archetype for blood pressure [Website: https://www.openehr.
      org/ckm/]   29
2.10 Hierarchy of different information objects in the ontology for
      health data of a remote health framework   36
2.11 Entities involved during a patient's visit to a doctor   37
2.12 Inheritance of the patient's history class   37
2.13 OWL file describing the inheritance of the history class . . .   38
2.14 OWL file describing the object properties of the treatment
      episode class   38
2.15 OWL file describing the data properties of the treatment
      episode class   39

4.1   Sensor on human body   66
4.2   Three-tier WBAN architecture   68
4.3   Inter-WBAN interference   75

5.1   Model of an ANN   91
5.2   Structure of an ANN   93
5.3   Step function   94
5.4   Sigmoid function   94
5.5   Hyperbolic tangent function   95
5.6   Architecture of a back propagation network   96
5.7   Set of points in 2D   100
5.8   Initialisation of clusters   101

5.9   Assignment of points to clusters   102
5.10   Assignment of points to clusters   103
5.11   A part of a decision tree   106
5.12   Samples of two classes that cannot be separated by a single
         straight line   108
5.13   The sample separated by two lines   109
5.14   Annual number of passengers in an airline   116

6.1   (a) Linear speedup, (b) Super-linear speedup, and (c) Sub-
         linear speedup   132
6.2   Execution of a parallel code - Amdahl's law   134
6.3   Shared memory multiprocessors   136
6.4   Distributed memory multicomputer   137
6.5   Distributed shared memory   138
6.6   A hierarchical hybrid architecture   139
6.7   GPU architecture [Source: [10]]   141
6.8   Memory organization in a GPU architecture [Source: [10]] .   142
6.9   Shared Address Space programming model   144
6.10   Message Passing programming model   145
6.11   A workflow of MapReduce program   146
6.12   MapReduce execution environment [Source: [6] [7]]   148
6.13   Hadoop architecture overview   149
6.14   YARN application execution   150
6.15   HDFS architecture   151
6.16   Apache Flume data model. [Source: https://flume.apache.org]   157
6.17   Apache Spark Streaming   158

7.1   MongoDB referencing relationship between data   170
7.2   MongoDB embedded documents   171
7.3   Cassandra column family [Source: [20]]   176
7.4   (a) Structure of a column, (b) Structure of a super column
         [Source: [20])   176
7.5   HBase table   179
7.6   Property Graph Model   182
7.7   Neo4j Graph Platform [Source: [6]]   183
7.8   A hierarchical data model for health data   184

Preface

With the advent of cloud computing and related technologies, eHealthcare is now in the focus of computer scientists and medical experts. According to Jeffrey P. Harrison, eHealthcare "is an all-encompassing term for the combined use of electronic information and communication technology in the health sector". The above definition assumes that information is transformed into electronic information, and then communication technology is used to transmit such information. So, health information first has to be converted and formatted into electronic health records for proper use. The electronic health information therefore may be made available wherever and whenever required. At the same time it has to be ensured that the information is reaching the rightful recipient. Care has to be taken so that it is not put into the wrong hands. Thus, eHealthcare aims at provisioning quality healthcare through efficient delivery using information and communication technologies. Wherever eHealthcare is possible, remote healthcare cannot be far behind. This means that patients in far off places (possibly remote locations) with negligible medical facilities will get access to doctors from urban areas. This is possible because of the penetration of communication technologies. Remote access to healthcare is therefore not a distant dream now, but has become feasible with the use of advanced communication technologies.

As a result of using eHealthcare, the interesting aspect that has drawn our attention is the generation of huge amounts of various data. Health data will contain data of a patient including his/her detailed personal information and health condition. Information regarding health condition may require X-ray reports, ECG reports, USG reports, or MRI reports, with other observations and reports of blood tests, to name a few. Thus, health data contains audio and video data, images. Health data will also include streaming sensor-generated data from continuous patient monitoring. This data has characteristics, like variety, velocity, and veracity, apart from being voluminous. Hence, health data is essentially, big data, or may be called Big Health Data. Big data is an evolving term to describe any voluminous amount of structured, semi-structured, and unstructured data that has the above properties along with many other properties. With so many properties, big data therefore also has the potential to be mined for information. It may be righfully observed that traditional relational databases may not be suitable for storing such big health data since the data may not always be confined to some structured format. Hence, NoSQL databases have been evolved to store such types of data. Several NoSQL database platforms developed and are in use. In order to improve the efficiency of information retrieval and also to improve the performance of the data analysis algorithms, distributed storage and distributed processing of the data is necessary. It is therefore apparent that the tasks of storage, management, and analysis of big health data are far from simple. Since the focus of this book is eHealthcare, and health data is considered to be secured and confidential, security of big data also becomes an issue. Thus, the issues regarding the handling of this big health data are many. Needless to say, the handling also needs to be different, since the nature of the data is very different from the data that have been handled so far.

The book focuses on the different aspects of handling big data in the healthcare domain. The book aims at providing insights into the eHealthcare domain from the perspective of big data. It attempts to provide a snapshot of the current scenario and existing techniques to meet the challenges. The chapters are organised in the following fashion: The first two chapters introduce the eHealthcare scenario and discuss the current state-of-the-art of storage and exchange of health records and health data models. Chapter 3 discusses the emerging concept of big data and explains why health data can be termed big data. The challenges involving handling issues of big data are also discussed in this chapter. The next three chapters of the book focus on the existing research challenges in big data acquisition, storage, management and analysis. Chapter 4 and Chapter 5 discuss techniques for data acquisition, data analysis, and data mining. Big data analytics has emerged as a new research area, and hence it is given focus in Chapter 5. Chapter 6 presents distributed data processing platforms and discusses several performance issues and performance improvement techniques. These are required for pursuing research in big data. Descriptions of some popular NoSQL platforms are included in Chapter 7. Chapter 7 also presents a case study of storing health data in one of the NoSQL databases. Chapter 8 discusses secured data storage and delivery along with privacy-preserving aspects. The focus is on eHealthcare applications, specifically, remote patient monitoring application.

This book can be used as a textbook for graduate students, and researchers will find it beneficial because the book covers handling of all aspects of big data in general and healthcare in particular. Graduate students can also use this book as a steppingstone for learning different aspects of big data. Each chapter of the book not only describes the current state of the art, but also attempts to indicate the research challenges. The book is aimed towards researchers who want to pursue research in handling big data issues in the healthcare domain. Researchers from different disciplines of engineering and technology will find this book helpful as it deals with issues regarding streaming data acquisition techniques. Medical professionals may also be interested in those chapters that deal with data analytics and data privacy.

Acknowledgements

All three authors have made equal contributions while writing this book. Additionally, some research scholars and postgraduate students of Jadavpur University have helped while preparing the manuscript. We would like to express our heartfelt thanks to everyone who has helped us in various capacities during the writing of this book. We thank our research scholars, Sayantani Saha, Sunanda Bose, Atrayee Gupta, Sriyanjana Adhikary, and Himadri Sekhar Ray, for their programming efforts in developing the remote healthcare system that serves as the backbone of this book. Part of the PhD research work of our doctoral student Poly Sil Sen and a portion of the Master of Engineering thesis work of the Masters degree student Kaushik Naguri have been used in the book, in Chapter 2 and Chapter 7. We thank them for their contribution. Thanks are due to the reviewers who provided us with detailed comments for the enrichment of the book. We thank all the people responsible for publication of this book right from the day of proposal.

Authors

Nandini Mukherjee received her PhD in Computer Science from the University of Manchester, United Kingdom, in 1999. She received a Commonwealth scholarship for her doctoral study in the UK. She completed the Masters in Computer Science and Engineering degree at Jadavpur University, Kolkata, India in 1991, and Bachelor of Engineering in Computer Science and Technology from Bengal Engineering College, Sibpur, India in 1987.

Since 1992, Nandini has been a faculty member in the Department of Computer Science and Engineering, Jadavpur University, Kolkata, India. Currently she is a professor in the department. She has served as director of the School of Mobile Computing and Communication, Jadavpur University for almost six years. Before joining Jadavpur University as a faculty member, Nandini also worked in industry for around three years.

Nandini Mukherjee is an active researcher in her chosen field. Her research interests are in the areas of high performance parallel computing, grid and cloud computing and wireless sensor networks. She has published more than 120 research papers in international peer-reviewed journals and proceedings of renowned international conferences. She also acted as a member of the technical program committees, organising committees and as reviewer for many international conferences and renowned journals. Nandini has acted as the lead investigator of many technical projects with social relevance. She is a senior member of IEEE and the IEEE Computer Society.

Sarmistha Neogy received her PhD degree in Engineering from Jadavpur University, Kolkata, India, in 2006. She obtained her Masters degree in Computer Science and Engineering and Bachelor degree in Computer Science and Engineering from Jadavpur University, in 1989 and 1987, respectively.

Sarmistha Neogy has served as a faculty member at University of Kalyani, University of Calcutta, before joining Jadavpur University in 2001. At present she is a professor in the Department of Computer Science and Engineering.

Sarmistha's research interests are in areas of fault tolerance in distributed systems, reliability and security in wireless and mobile systems, and wireless sensor networks. She is a senior member of IEEE and the IEEE Computer Society. She has publications in international journals and proceedings of international conferences. She also acts as a member in the technical program committee of international conferences and has reviewed for international journals. She has delivered tutorial lectures in international conferences.

Samiran Chattopadhyay is a professor in the Department of Information Technology, Jadavpur University. He has served as the head of the department for more than twelve years and as the Joint Director of the School of Mobile Computing and Communication since its inception. A graduate, post-graduate and gold medalist from Indian Institute of Technology, Kharagpur he received his PhD Degree from Jadavpur University. Samiran has two decades of experience in serving renowned industry houses such as Computer Associates, Interra Systems India, Agilent, and Motorola, in the capacity of technical consultant. He led the development of an open-source C++ infrastructure and tool set for reconfigurable computing, released under the GNU GPL 3.0 license. Samiran has visited several Universities in the United Kingdom as a visiting professor. He has been working on algorithms for security, bio informatics, distributed and mobile Computing, and middleware. He has authored and edited several books and book chapters. Samiran acted as a programme chair, organising chair, and IPC member of over 20 international conferences. He has published more than 120 papers in reputed journals and international peer reviewed conferences.

1

Introduction

CONTENTS

1.1   What Is eHealth? 2
1.2   eHealth Technologies 3
1.3   eHealth Applications 4
     1.3.1   Health Informatics 5
     1.3.2   mHealth 5
     1.3.3   Telehealth 6
1.4   eHealth and Big Data 8
1.5   Issues and Challenges 9
1.6   Chapter Notes 11

The Health-For-All policy of the World Health Organisation (WHO) envisions securing the health and well being of people around the world. The policy was introduced in the 1970s, and based on this policy, new strategies have been adopted in the subsequent years. The policy forms the basis of the primary healthcare strategy of the World Health Organisation, aiming at promoting health, human dignity, and enhanced quality of life.

Gradually, over the years, the role of technologies in the healthcare sector has been perceived. In 1997, an international consultation convened by WHO prepared input on "telematics" for the health-for-all policy of WHO, targeting global health development in the twenty-first century. The report generated through this consultation suggests appropriate use of health telematics in the overall policy and strategy of WHO for major public health purposes [9]. In subsequent years, considering the huge impact of information and communication technologies in healthcare services, the *World Health Assembly* the decision-making body of WHO adopted a resolution in 2005 to formulate an eHealth strategy for WHO. In this resolution, eHealth is defined as the *"cost-effective and secure use of information and communication technologies in support of health and health-related fields, including healthcare services, health surveillance, health literature, and health education"*. In its Geneva meeting in 2005, the WHO executive board recommended to the World Health Assembly, inter alia, "to continue the expansion to Member States of mechanisms such as the Health Academy which promote health awareness and healthy lifestyles through eLearning". While adopting the resolution, the executive board also considered the *Millennium Development Goals (MDGs)*, which were estab-

1

lished following a millennium summit of the United Nations in 2000. The monitoring framework for the MDGs consisted of a list of 18 targets and 48 indicators. Target 18 in this list clearly directs to "make available the benefits of new technologies, especially information and communications" for sustainable development.

1.1   What Is eHealth?

In the report produced by the Executive Board of WHO, eHealth is defined as *the use of information and communication technologies locally and at a distance to present a unique opportunity for the development of public health* [1]. The report also observes that the strengthening of health systems through eHealth reinforces fundamental human rights by improving equity, solidarity, quality of life, and quality of care.

G. Eysenbach defines eHealth as *"an emerging field in the intersection of medical informatics, public health and business, referring to health services and information delivered or enhanced through the Internet and related technologies. In a broader sense, the term characterizes not only a technical development, but also a state-of-mind, a way of thinking, an attitude, and a commitment for networked, global thinking, to improve healthcare locally, regionally, and worldwide by using information and communication technology"* [3].

On the other hand, the European Commission defines eHealth as *"the use of modern information and communication technologies to meet needs of citizens, patients, healthcare professionals, healthcare providers, as well as policy makers"* [7].

According to the description provided by the European Commission [2], eHealth or digital health and care covers the following areas:

- Information and data sharing between patients and health service providers, hospitals, health professionals, and health information networks

- Electronic health records

- Telemedicine services

- Portable patient-monitoring devices

- Operating room scheduling software, and

- Robotised surgery

In 2016, WHO published a survey report on how eHealth can support universal health coverage (UHC) [4]. The survey was conducted in the member states, and a total of 125 countries participated in this survey. WHO observes that provisioning eHealth services can range from gathering and disseminating information to keeping citizens healthy, supporting public health in communities, developing care and support systems in health facilities, and from all such systems, collecting data which is needed for management and the policymakers. According to the report, there is an upward trend in the adoption of eHealth. The adoption of eHealth policy has accelerated since 2005 and almost 58% of countries now have an eHealth strategy.

1.2 eHealth Technologies

Most eHealth solutions are based on five key technologies. These technologies include:

- Websites: Most of the early eHealth solutions are web-based. These solutions are accessed from all over the world for various purposes. For example, in the Netherlands, psychologists prescribe web-based modules to help patients to overcome anxiety disorders or to provide care for the patients with autism. Websites can also be used to deal with many other problems, such as alcohol addiction. In developed countries, websites are used for storing health records (nowadays in the form of electronic health records or EHRs) of patients with chronic diseases, so that this data can be used by the healthcare professionals for future reference.

- Videoconferencing: Patients may want to consult remotely located doctors using videoconferencing. Doctors may also want to visualise the injuries, burns, or rashes on a patient's body, so that they can prescribe medication more precisely.

- Mobile Apps: Several mobile apps have been developed during the last few years. Some of these are used by the patients for taking care of their own health. These include helping the patients learn relaxation skills, monitoring proper diets, making sure they get enough exercise etc. Apps can also be used by healthcare workers; for example to assist nurses in administering the right medication, etc.

- Wearable Devices: The wearable technologies are used to gather clinical parameters from a patient's body and transfer the measured parameters to apps which are used to monitor the patients' health. Many of these wearables can monitor sleep and movement of the patients, and vitals like heart rate, etc., during the entire day.

- Virtual Reality: In some countries, virtual reality (VR) is used within a hospital environment for helping patients to psychologically overcome certain problems. An example of such use of virtual reality is the treatment of people with a fear of flying by exposing them to flight in a VR environment.

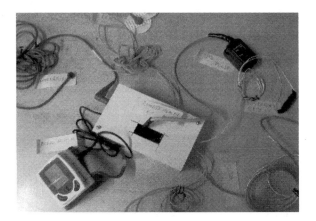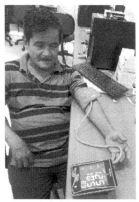

FIGURE 1.1: eHealth sensors and medical IoT development platform

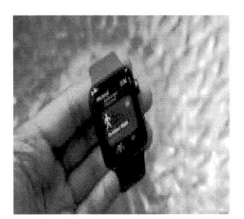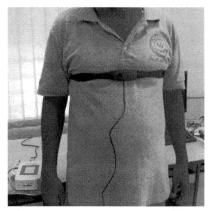

FIGURE 1.2: Wearable technology

1.3 eHealth Applications

In the previous sections, the areas covered under eHealth and the associated technologies were mentioned. This section describes recent advances in those areas.

1.3.1 Health Informatics

The term *health informatics* focuses on the actions related to acquiring, storing, retrieving, and using healthcare information to provide better care to patients. This is an evolving specialisation which is based on information and communication technologies.

On the other hand, health information technology or *Health IT* refers to the technology tools which are used by the caregivers (physicians and nurses), administrators, patients, and other stakeholders for storage, analysis, and sharing of health information. Such tools include electronic health records (EHR), healthcare apps, prescription generation apps, and several others. The Centers for Disease Control and Prevention of the United States distinguishes between the two terms, mentioning that informatics is "the science, the how and why, behind health IT". With the help of health informatics, the concepts, theories, and practices are applied to real-life situations [5].

During the last few years, access to medical and health information has exponentially increased, and variety of health information resources have been made available. Alongside these, a number of self-management and risk assessment tools are also available over the Internet. Surveys conducted in United States show that three-fourths of the American population consult online resources to obtain health information [8].

Today a number of tools (generally web-based) are available to store and retrieve medical information of patients, including past histories, medications, treatments, insurance policies etc. for future use. However, in this context, the major challenge is that this data is often distributed on computing resources across different clinics, specialists, institutions, etc. Extracting knowledge from such distributed data storage systems require efficient data handling and processing techniques. Some tools are available which allow the patients to assume greater responsibilities and manage their own personal information. These tools assure better quality of healthcare for the patients by increasing accuracy, completeness, accessibility, and portability of health records.

Web-based services are also used to enhance communication between patients and care providers. Although various synchronous and asynchronous communication technologies, such as emails, text messaging, interactive video chats, etc. are already in use by patients and caregivers (doctors, nurses, insurance companies, etc.), the adoption of online services is relatively slow. It has been observed that patients are often concerned about the security and privacy of the data while using offline or online communication technologies.

1.3.2 mHealth

In a survey conducted by WHO Global Observatory for eHealth in 2015, mobile health or mHealth was defined as *the services or applications which are provided and/or accessed using mobile phones, personal digital assistants*

(PDAs) or other types of patient monitoring devices and wireless devices for the purpose of medical and public health practices.

mHealth increases patients' access to and provision of health services for citizens; in particular, the underserved communities, and people living in remote areas and in areas where there is no or little infrastructure to support traditional healthcare services. Even in the absence of traditional communication network, i.e., wired or wireless networks, mHealth services can be made available with the help of mobile communications technology.

Use of mobile devices has increased rapidly across most countries in the world. The growth has been particularly faster in the developing countries. The number of subscriptions for mobile broadband has also increased rapidly to cover 86% of the inhabitants in developed countries and 39% in the developing countries, surpassing global fixed broadband subscriptions in 2008 and fixed telephone lines in 2012 [4].

The most common digital health applications for mHealth include: education and awareness, diagnostic and treatment support, disease and epidemic outbreak tracking, and healthcare supply-chain management. Other important applications are remote data collection, remote monitoring, healthcare worker telecommunication and training, telehealth/telemedicine and chronic disease management. Table 1.1 [1] lists a set of mHealth services as specified by WHO [4] for the survey conducted in 2015.

Wearable devices are often connected with mHealth services to facilitate disease diagnosis remotely. One such example is the study initiated at the University of California in San Diego that integrates mHealth wearables, such as Apple Watch and Android Wear, with an AI platform, to detect early signs of diabetes from the heart rate and step counts of a patient.

Another study conducted by the American Medical Group Foundation attempts to improve hypertension detection and control using a smartphone-connected automatic blood pressure (BP) device to record the blood pressure reading of a patient and storing it on his or her smart device. This reading is then automatically sent to the caregiver for reviewing. The caregiver thus can efficiently titrate medications, educate the patient about lifestyle, and advise visits to doctors when necessary. Other devices, such as ECG and blood glucose monitors can be used in a similar manner.

1.3.3   Telehealth

Interaction between a healthcare provider and a patient when the two are separated by distance is termed telehealth. The interaction may take place synchronously or asynchronously. Examples of synchronous interaction are telephone conversations or interactions over a video link in real time. On the other hand, asynchronous interaction implies store-and-forward type commu-

---

[1]Reprinted from Global diffusion of eHealth: Making universal health coverage achievable: Report of the third global survey on eHealth: Global Observatory for eHealth – 2016.

TABLE 1.1: Types of mHealth Programmes

Service	Description
Communication between individuals and health services	
Health call centres or health care telephone helplines	Healthcare advice and triage provided by trained personnel and pre-recorded messages; accessible on mobile phones or fixed lines.
Emergency toll-free telephone services	Free telephone hotlines for health emergencies provided by trained personnel and pre-recorded messages, and linked to response systems; accessible on mobile phones or fixed lines.
Communication between health services and individuals	
Treatment adherence	Reminder messages provided by health services to patients aimed at achieving medication adherence using mobile ICT; messages can be text, voice, or multimedia.
Reminder to attend appointments	Reminder messages provided by health services to patients to make or attend an appointment using mobile ICT; message can be text, voice, or multimedia.
Community mobilisation/health promotion campaigns	Health promotion campaigns conducted using mobile ICT to raise the awareness of target groups. Messages conveying information can be text, voice or multimedia.
Consultation between healthcare professionals	
Mobile telehealth	Consultation between healthcare practitioners or between practitioners and patients using mobile ICT.
Intersectoral communication in emergencies	
Emergency management systems	Response to and management of emergency and disaster situations using mobile ICT.
Heath monitoring and surveillance	
Health surveys	Data collection, management, and reporting of health surveys using mobile ICT. May involve any combination of networked mobile devices.
Surveillance	Routine, emergency, and targeted data collection, management, and reporting for public health surveillance using mobile ICT. May involve any combination of networked mobile devices.
Patient monitoring	Data capture and transmission for monitoring a variety of conditions in a range of settings using mobile ICT.
Access to information and education for healthcare professionals	
Access to information, resources, databases and tools	Access to health sciences literature, resources, and databases using mobile ICT.
Clinical decision support systems	Access to decision support systems using mobile ICT.
Electronic patient information	Access to electronic patient information (such as EHR/EMR, laboratory results, X-rays, etc.) using mobile ICT.
mLearning	Access to online educational resources using mobile ICT.

nication, i.e., a query is submitted and the answer is provided later. Email is an example of this type of interaction.

WHO defines telehealth as follows [4]: *"the delivery of healthcare services, where patients and providers are separated by distance. Telehealth uses ICT for the exchange of information for the diagnosis and treatment of diseases and injuries, research and evaluation, and for the continuing education of health professionals. Telehealth can contribute to achieving universal health coverage by improving access for patients to quality, cost-effective, health services wherever they may be. It is particularly valuable for those in remote areas, vulnerable groups and aging populations."*

Telehealth is also defined as the use of electronic information and telecommunication technologies to remotely support and promote clinical healthcare, patient and professional health-related education, and public health and health administration [6]. Technologies used for telehealth services include videoconferencing, the Internet, store-and-forward imaging, streaming media, and terrestrial and wireless communications.

Telehealth is particularly useful for management of long term health conditions, including Chronic Obstructive Pulmonary Disease (COPD), Chronic Heart Failure (CHF), Diabetes, and Epilepsy. Vital signs, such as blood pressure, are monitored and transmitted via a telephone line to a telehealth monitoring centre or a healthcare professional. The data is checked against a set of parameters set by the healthcare professional or doctor. Whenever a vital sign is outside the 'normal' range, alerts are generated.

A commonly used term is *telemedicine*, which has been in use for a long time. Telemedicine is concerned with the clinical application of technology. On the other hand, telehealth is used in a broader context. It is not just a specific clinical service, but rather "a collection of means or methods to enhance care delivery and education" (according to the federal network of telehealth resource centres). Telehealth is also not just traditional diagnostic and monitoring activities. It also includes consumer and professional education in the health sector.

1.4   eHealth and Big Data

As is evident from the previous discussion, eHealthcare initiatives are primarily aimed towards access, quality, affordability, lowering the disease burden, and efficient monitoring of health entitlements to citizens. An integrated approach to medical and health informatics, translational bioinformatics, sensor informatics, and imaging informatics together with different aspects of personalized information will immensely benefit the eHealthcare projects . The information may be obtained from a diverse range of data sources, covering both structured and unstructured formats, including imaging, clinical diagnosis, continuous physiological monitoring, genomics, and so on.

As is evident, data will be generated in huge amount and in diverse formats. These data have to be stored properly for a number of tasks, namely, prescription generation by medical practitioners, necessary actions to be taken by healthcare professionals (say, nurses), awareness of personal health condition (patient), research purposes, and marketing, to name a few. None other than big data is able to take care of this mammoth task. Simply speaking, *big data* may be considered to be this huge amount of diverse type of data taken all together.

Going by the recent advances in technologies, it is only expected that *big data* will take the lead henceforth. The nature of data being different, existing storage and database types, data accessing policies and techniques, techniques of protecting the data, algorithms for analysis, parameters to be considered for analysis and inferences will not be same as earlier. Hence, researchers, designers, and developers have already joined hands and have come up with new ideas and technologies and implementations.

It may also be observed here that eHealthcare has come to stay. This is because the needs of users have evolved over time. People are now becoming more aware about their rights. Stakeholders including patients, doctors, healthcare professionals, researchers, pathologists, and pharmaceutical companies have their own requirements as well as responsibilities. Patients want to be abreast of their health condition, whereas doctors also want to have the latest information about a patient. Similarly, researchers may be interested in different analytics using this huge data. Pharmaceutical companies will be interested in knowing the market for their drugs, and hence, will indirectly depend on other sources of information. People also want to exercise their rights properly. They are keen to be part of experimental systems, too. Patients themselves may sign up for new drug trials, because they want to experience the benefit for themselves on their own. Each of the above-mentioned activities is generating data continuously. So eHealth is the only way out. And with the massive ever-growing data, big data is its only means of expression!!

1.5   Issues and Challenges

We mentioned earlier that a huge amount of data is generated from eHealth solutions. The data has the properties of big data, i.e., not only volume, but variety, velocity, and veracity. We discuss the properties of health data in detail in Chapter 3. Handling such a huge amount of data is a real challenge.

The data is generated from various sources and stored in different formats. Standards must be evolved for sharing and exchanging these data among different organisations, so that the actual meaning of the data is not lost. Further, although many parts of this data are generally structured, there are other parts which are semi-structured or do not have any structure at all. Therefore, modeling and storing such data for efficient retrieval is another challenge.

With the rapid increase in the use of wearables and mobile devices embedded with sensors, a large number of clinical parameters can be collected continuously in real time. It may not always be possible to transfer such a large volume of data from the edge devices (mobiles, sensors, etc.) to the remote data centres due to low bandwidth, transmission cost, interference, and other issues. Thus, data acquisition is also a challenge which needs to be dealt with.

Processing this data and extracting useful knowledge is necessary for better treatment of patients or for general improvement of community health. New algorithms have evolved for processing the data, and also, new technologies have been invented for improving the performance of processing the data.

Finally, health data is sensitive, and therefore, the security and privacy of data must be given the utmost priority. As the data is transmitted over the non-dependable Internet, security mechanisms for the network should be strengthened. The stored data also needs to be secured.

Figure 1.3 highlights some of the issues and challenges which will be discussed in this book, in the subsequent chapters.

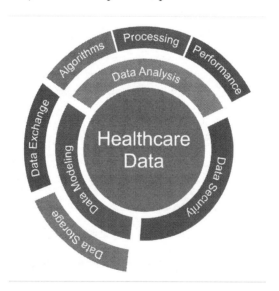

FIGURE 1.3: Issues in eHealth data

1.6   Chapter Notes

The purview of this book is issues and challenges of big data in eHealthcare. Big data is viewed from different perspectives in the different chapters of this book.

The tone of the book is set with the introduction to the eHealthcare scenario. Discussions about the current state of the art of health-record format along with health data storage and health data models follow. The concept of big data and its nuances are also taken up. Health data is found to possess big data properties. The role of big data in eHealthcare is discussed. Chapters of this book focus on techniques of data acquisition, storage models, and evolving concept of databases for big data. Research challenges faced by health big data analytics and methods of handling them are also included in the book. Computation models for handling big data are discussed. One of the most important issues that big data faces is security. Security and privacy may be considered to be two sides of the same coin. Secure storage and privacy preserving data access are dealt with in this book.

References

[1] Executive Board 115. eHealth: Report by the Secretariat. Executive Board 115th session, provisional agenda item 4.13 EB115/39, World Health Organization, December 2004.

[2] European Commission. eHealth : Digital health and care. Website: `https://ec.europa.eu/health/ehealth/overview_en`.

[3] G. Eysenbach. What is eHealth? *Journal of Medical Internet Research*, 3(2), 2001.

[4] Global Observatory for eHealth. *Global diffusion of eHealth: Making universal health coverage achievable: Report of the third global survey on eHealth*. World Health Organization, Website: `www.who.int/goe/publications/global_diffusion/en/`, 2016.

[5] USF Health. What is Health Informatics? Website: `https://www.usfhealthonline.com`.

[6] Health Resources and Services Administration Federal Office of Rural Health Policy. Website: `http://www.hrsa.gov/ruralhealth/telehealth/`.

[7] Innovatemedtec. eHealth. Website: `https://innovatemedtec.com/digital-health/ehealth`.

[8] M. L. A. Lustria, S. A. Smith, and C. C. Hinnant. Exploring digital divides: an examination of eHealth technology use in health information seeking, communication and personal health information management in the USA. *Health Informatics Journal*, 17(3):224–243, 2011.

[9] WHO Group Consultation on Health Telematics (1997: Geneva, Switzerland). A health telematics policy in support of WHO's Health-for-all strategy for global health development. Technical Report WHO/DGO/98.1, World Health Organization, Website: `http://www.who.int/iris/handle/10665/63857`, December 1998.

2

Electronic Health Records

CONTENTS

2.1	Introduction	13
2.2	Electronic Health Records	14
2.3	EHR Standards	16
	2.3.1 ISO 13606	17
	2.3.2 HL7	18
	2.3.3 OpenEHR	23
2.4	Adoption of EHR Standards	30
2.5	Ontology-based Approaches	32
	2.5.1 Developing an Ontology	33
	2.5.2 Ontologies for EHR	33
	2.5.3 Ontologies in Healthcare	34
2.6	Chapter Notes	35

2.1 Introduction

A major concern for developing eHealth services is how to develop an effective data model, and how to store data for efficient retrieval by eHealth services. The health data collected by the eHealth service delivery framework is required to be stored following a schema which may be static or dynamic, or, in special cases, may be static with the option to be dynamic. In order to develop an integrated approach to storing and maintaining health data, it is necessary to follow national and international standards of storing electronic health records (EHR).

The present scenarios for eHealth applications demonstrate that health data has properties like volume, variety, velocity, and veracity to be treated as big data. The four properties are observed as follows:

- Health data is generated in large volume. It includes demographic and family history details of patients, their visits to doctors, treatment plans, physical investigation reports, and clinical parameters monitoring data from sensors. Thus, the data generated through any eHealth application is voluminous.

- Health data complies with the second big data property, i.e., variety, because health data needs to be stored in different forms, like textual data (patient history, measurement of clinical parameters), image data (ECG, X-ray reports), audio data (sound of heartbeat), etc.

- While performing continuous monitoring of a patient, data is generated continuously from the sensors or *Wireless Body Area Network* (WBAN) attached to the patients' bodies. Continuous data generation and requirement of fast processing of this huge amount of data account for the velocity. There is a requirement for storing and analyzing this data in appropriate manner.

- Also, the veracity property holds in the case of health data due to its uncertainty while measuring using sensors, and at times, for several other reasons, such as inability of the patients to communicate properly and lack of thorough observations by the caregivers.

Health data is complicated in structure — some parts of it are structured and other parts are unstructured. It is observed by many researchers that different types of data structures are to be used as parts of health data.

In this chapter we introduce *Electronic Health Records* (EHR) and *Electronic Medical Records* (EMR), which are defined for storing the health information of patients, and discuss the various standards of storing such information.

2.2   Electronic Health Records

An *Electronic Health Record* or EHR is defined as "a repository of information regarding the health status of a subject of care in computer processable form, stored and transmitted securely, and accessible by multiple authorized users. It has a standardized or commonly agreed logical information model which is independent of EHR systems. Its primary purpose is the support of continuing, efficient and quality integrated healthcare and it contains information which is retrospective, concurrent, and prospective" [4].

Electronic health records are considered to be a summary of various electronic medical records which are generated during clinical encounters. Thus, an electronic health record of a person is defined as an aggregation of all electronic medical records of the person from his or her very first entry into the healthcare system until today. It is recommended that all records be preserved during the lifetime of the individual. EHRs can contain a patient's medical history, diagnoses, medications, treatment plans, immunisation dates, allergies, radiology images, and laboratory and test results. Effectively, EHRs allow access to evidence-based tools that providers can use to make decisions about a patient's care and automate and streamline provider workflow.

Difference between EHR and EMR

Electronic Health Records (EHR) and *Electronic Medical Records* (EMR) are often used interchangeably. In fact, some confusion arises regarding whether an EHR differs from an EMR or not. However, in the present circumstances, the term EHR is referenced more frequently and considered to encompass more information compared to an EMR. Electronic medical records contain only clinical data of a patient, whereas electronic health records go beyond that to focus on the broader, total health of each patient [10] [23].

Thus, an EMR contains the medical and treatment history of the patients generated in one single clinic/hospital. The information in EMRs therefore is normally used only within the boundary of the clinic/hospital and does not move beyond that.

On the other hand, EHRs are designed for use within a wider boundary, i.e., beyond the health organisation where such data is originally collected and compiled. EHRs are generated to share information between several healthcare providers, such as clinics, hospitals, laboratories, and specialists, so that they are updated by all such organisations involved in the patient's care and store information from all of them. The EHR data "can be created, managed, and consulted by authorised clinicians and staff across more than one healthcare organization." (as stated by The National Alliance for Health Information Technology (NAHIT) in the United States of America). It is therefore possible to move the information simultaneously with a patient across hospitals, states, and countries.

EHR System

While an EHR contains the medical and treatment histories of patients, an *EHR system* (EHR-S) may be built to contain information beyond standard clinical data and can be inclusive of a broader view of the information related to the healthcare facilities for the patients.

The EHR-S can be considered as an integration of patient information systems. It generates a data stream and provides support for health data analysis, policymaking, controlling the overall disease burden of the country, and performing research in social perspective. The EHR-S includes the network that links databases, interfaces, order entry, electronic communication systems, and the clinical servers (ISO TC 215, ISO/TR 20514:2005) [4]. An EHR system also contains security, privacy, and legal data [9].

The EHR System or EHR-S is defined to include [5]:

1. Longitudinal collection of electronic health information for and about persons, where health information is defined as information pertaining to the health of an individual or healthcare provided to an individual;

2. Immediate electronic access to individual-level and population-level information by authorised, and only authorised, users;

3. Provision of knowledge and decision-support that enhance the quality, safety, and efficiency of patient care; and

4. Support of efficient processes for healthcare delivery.

Benefits of EHR

A personal health record is implemented as a documentation of any form of patient information, which includes medical history, medicines, allergies, visits to the doctors, and vaccinations.

With fully functional EHRs, all caregivers (doctors, nurses, management personnel) have ready access to the latest information, allowing more coordinated care for the patients. Patients themselves should be able to view, carry, amend, annotate, or maintain the data. Thus, the information gathered by the primary care provider can inform the emergency department clinician about the patient's life threatening allergy, so that care can be taken even if the patient is unable to share such information. A patient can view his or her own record and observe the trend of the lab results over the last year. A specialist can view the recent pathological or other tests to avoid any duplication. The notes regarding the patient's treatment in a hospital can help to inform the follow-up care and enable the patient to move smoothly from one care provider to another.

2.3   EHR Standards

So far, many standards of EHR have been defined. These standards try to provide guidelines for storing, manipulating and using clinical information in a suitable manner, so that they can be retrieved efficiently at the time of need. Three main standard bodies are currently active in the international standards domain for directly defining and modifying the EHR standards. These organisations are (i) International Standards Organization (ISO), (ii) *(Comité Européen de Normalisation)* — the European Committee for Standardization (CEN), and (iii) Health Level 7 (HL7). Another popular and efficient EHR standard, openEHR, is gradually evolving with the support from a virtual community.

In addition to the above organisations, the American Society for Testing and Materials (ASTM) International provided an EHR standard with an objective of defining the attributes necessary for successful implementation of an EHR [5]. The standard covered all types of healthcare services containing acute care in hospitals, nursing homes, specialty care, care at home, and in ambulances, etc. The attributes were defined to include description of patients, identifying information for patients, legal permissions, treatment plans, documentation for actions taken, etc. Important relations that exist among data retrieved from various sources were also described in this standard. However, the standard was withdrawn in March 2017 without replacement. The rationale behind the withdrawal decision has been its limited use by industries.

In the remaining part of this section, the emerging standards, ISO 13606, HL7, and openEHR are discussed in detail.

2.3.1 ISO 13606

The European standards organization, CEN recommended a standard for EHR, called the Electronic Health Record Communication (EN 13606). The standard is not intended to specify the internal architecture or database design of EHR systems or components. Rather, it defines an information architecture for communicating part or all of the EHR of a single subject of care (patient). Thus, the standard extends support to the interoperability of systems and components that need to communicate (stored, retrieved, and exchanged) EHR data via electronic messages or as distributed objects.

The standard offered by CEN, known as CEN EN13606, has five parts: (1) Reference Model, (2) Archetype Interchange Specification, (3) Reference Archetypes and Term Lists, (4) Security Attributes and (5) Exchange Model [17]. Later, it has become internationally ratified by ISO and has been recognised as the **ISO/EN 13606 standard**.

The ISO standard recognises that there is a need for *semantic interoperability* of data along with *syntactic interoperability* . Syntactic interoperability assures that two or more systems are capable of communicating and exchanging data by using the same data formats or communication protocols. Some well-known data exchange formats are XML and JSON. Most standards guarantee syntactic interoperability, whereas semantic interoperability indicates that the system should have the ability to automatically interpret the information exchanged meaningfully and accurately, so that the end-users are benefited. Syntactic interoperability guarantees the exchange of the structure of the data, but carries no assurance that the meaning will be interpreted identically by all parties [15]. On the other hand, semantic interoperability is the ability to interpret the information shared within the systems as efficiently as necessary for the formally defined domain concepts [7]. To achieve semantic interoperability, the participating bodies must accept a common information exchange reference model. Thus, the contents of the information exchange requests must be defined without any ambiguity.

In the field of health informatics, achieving semantic interoperability is important. The semantic interoperability (along with syntactic interoperability) is enforced by the ISO/EN 13606 standard by defining a dual model architecture. The dual model architecture structures information through a *reference model* and knowledge through *archetypes*, thereby ensuring a clear separation between information and knowledge. The reference model contains the basic entities for representing any information of the EHR, while the latter, i.e., archetypes, provide formal definitions of clinical information models, such as discharge report, glucose measurement, or family history. Thus, the reference model provides the building blocks, i.e., the generic classes and structures for the EHR. On the other hand, archetypes define valid combinations of the building blocks with specific meanings. Archtypes are not used for holding any data, but rather to define a template for the data.

ISO 13606 Reference Model contains [1]:

- A set of classes to represent clinical information. Any annotation in an EHR must be an instance of one of these classes. ISO 13606 defines six clinical classes: *folder, composition, section, entry, cluster,* and *element.* Additionally, it includes a class to represent an *EHRextract*, which covers use cases including EHR system communication, other clinical content messaging, and EHR system synchronisation.

- A set of classes to represent context information to be attached to an EHR annotation, including versioning information.

- A set of classes to describe demographic data.

- A set of classes to represent data types.

ISO/EN 13606 forms a subset of the OpenEHR standard. At the same time, ISO/EN 13606 offers a partial alignment with HL7 Clinical Document Architecture (CDA).

2.3.2   HL7

HL7 has created *messaging standards*, as well as standards for Continuity of Care Documents (CCD), and Clinical Document Architecture (CDA) files [26] [28]. These standards describe how clinical data are exchanged between different EHR systems. Unlike ASTM, which works in various domains, the HL7 International working group works in the specific domains of clinical and administrative data. Some of the standards of HL7 International are also equivalent to ISO TC-215 standards. The scope of TC-215 is standardisation in the field of health informatics to facilitate health applications for the interchange and use of health-related data, information, and knowledge, coherently and consistently, to support and enable all aspects of the health system. ISO TC-215 adopts specific HL7 International standards, and also works with HL7 International to jointly develop or modify HL7 standards.

The term 'Level Seven' in HL7 refers to the highest layer of the OSI model (Open Systems Interconnection) of communication and networking standards of ISO, i.e., the application layer. The application layer, i.e. the seventh layer in the OSI model, defines the data to be exchanged, the timing of the interchange, and the communication of certain errors to the application. This layer also supports functions like security checks, participant identification, availability checks, exchange mechanism negotiations, and data exchange structuring.

Version 1.0 of HL7 was published in 1988, followed by Version 2.0 in 1989.

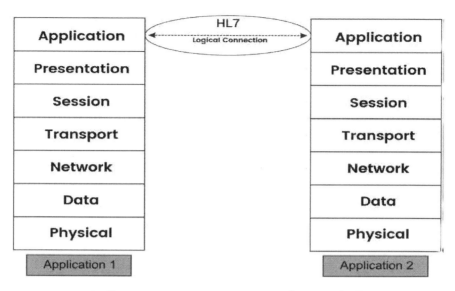

FIGURE 2.1: HL7 and OSI layers [Source: [18]]

Later, a number of releases of Versions 2.x were published, and finally an initial publication of Version 3 was made in 2005.

HL7 International has over one hundred products. However, the most widely used is *HL7 Electronic Data Exchange in Healthcare Environments.* This is a messaging standard enabling the development of implementation guides to facilitate healthcare applications, to exchange clinical and administrative data in a predefined fashion.

In HL7, a message is event-driven and includes a specific workflow. It can include bi-directional flow of data. For example, a 'lab test may be ordered' in one direction, and in response to this message, a 'test report may be communicated' in the reverse direction.

In addition to message exchange standards, HL7 developed the following standards:

1. *Arden Syntax,* which provides specification covering the sharing of computerised health knowledge bases among personnel, information systems, and institutions;

2. GELLO — *Standard Expression Language* for decision support;

3. Version 2.x XML, i.e., an XML encoding of HL7 International messages;

4. *HL7 Version 3 Clinical Document Architecture (CDA),* which provides a facility for clinical summary information transfer as structured parseable documents;

5. *Electronic Health Record System (EHR-S) Functional Model;*

6. *Personal Health Record System (PHR-S) Functional Model;*

7. *Services* related to a *Services Oriented Architecture.*

HL7 Version 3

The Version 3 standard, as opposed to Version 2, is based on a formal methodology (the HL7 Development Framework) and object-oriented principles. The information is organised into classes having attributes, and the classes have associations with other classes. Version 3 develops a single, common *reference information model* (RIM) that can be used across all products of HL7, enabling the care providers to document the actions taken to treat a patient. Such actions include a request or order for a test, reporting the test results, creating a diagnosis based on test results, and prescribing treatment based on the diagnosis. Thus, every happening in the *reference information model* is an **Act**. Acts are procedures, observations, medications, supply, registration, etc. Acts are related through **ActRelationships**, which may be composition, precondition, revision, support, etc. In the RIM, persons, organisations, materials, places, devices, etc., are treated as **Entities**. Entities play some **Roles**, such as patient, provider, practitioner, specimen, and employee. Roles participate in acts and the **Participation** is defined as the context of an act, such as author, performer, subject, location, etc. The definitions of the above-mentioned classes are given below [28]:

- **Act** — an action in the healthcare domain of HL7. Whenever necessary, intentional actions are taken in healthcare (or in any other profession or business). An instance of an act is stored as a record. Act definitions (master files), orders, plans, and performance records (events) are all represented by an instance of an act.

- **Act Relationship** — Two acts are related to each other through some kind of relationships. Examples of these relationships can be 'compositional', 'reference' and 'succeeds'.

- **Entity** — An entity is a physical thing or organisation, or a group of physical things. A physical thing is anything that has extent in space, or mass. It does not include information structures, electronic medical records, messages, data structures, etc.

- **Role** — It is a socially expected behavior pattern usually determined by the status of an individual in a particular society. For people, role is usually positions, jobs, and a function performed especially in a particular operation or process.

- **Role Link** — Role link is a relationship between two entity roles. For example, a physician's relationship with an organisation and a pa-

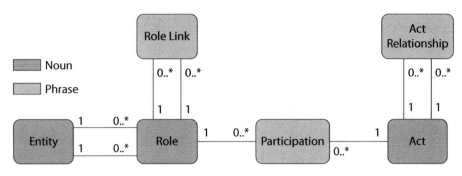

FIGURE 2.2: Core classes of RIM

tient's relationship with the organisation may be linked to express the relationship between the patient and physician.

- **Participation** — Participation exists only within the scope of the acts. There may be multiple participants in an act. Each participant is an entity in a role. Thus, role signifies competence while participation signifies performance.

Figure 2.2 depicts the core classes of RIM. In the figure, nouns are typically actions or entities, whereas phrases are the relationships, i.e., the bindings between them.

In the reference information model, *concept domain* defines concepts to represent an attribute in a particular design, *code system* provides a set of coded concepts, *value set* selects a subset of the coded concepts and *binding* asserts that a particular value set satisfies the domain.

The entity diagram, role diagram, and the participation and act diagram of HL7 reference information model are shown in Figures 2.3, 2.4, and 2.5, respectively.

Based on the reference model within Version 3, and a set of tools provided by HL7, a process can produce a simple common, sharable resource for patients, standard clinical documents for various uses, voluminous and rich sets of information containing electronic claims, clinical trial data and clinical genomics information structures.

Version 3 messages are generated and sent from the sending application to the receiving application using industry standard technologies for implementation and transport, such as XML, SOAP, and WSDL. The messages support activities, such as person registry queries and responses, request/response for insurance authorisation, notification of an adverse event (to the public health

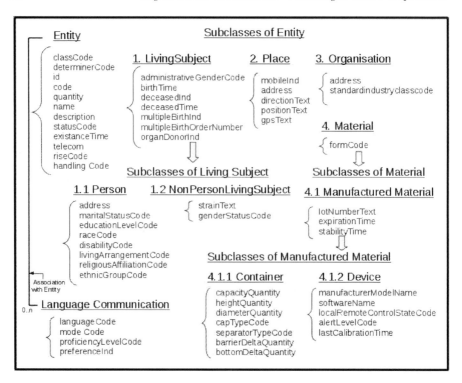

FIGURE 2.3: Entity class and its subclasses [Source: [28]]

authority), notification of a finalised lab result, pharmacy order fulfillment request/response, notification of care transfer, etc.

The Clinical Document Architecture (CDA) of Version 3 provides a document standard, i.e., a standard for document sharing. CDA facilitates document exchange within and between medical institutions. CDA documents can be transmitted by encapsulating them within a Version 3 message. However, these documents can also exist in non-messaging contexts. These documents are more oriented towards readability by people, not machines. CDA can be used to bring a patient's clinical documents into a patient-centric EHR. It is often a collection of information about an encounter and can be digitally signed. CDA provides an approved standard way to exchange dictated, scanned, or electronic reports of a patient between various health information systems and platforms. CDA facilitates the storage and management of clinical data and the context driven analysis of data, and increases data reusability.

Although HL7 allows interoperability, this data model is not sufficient to cover all actors and actions of a clinical system. HL7 RIM is not prepared to be an EHR information model. It contains terminologies that can work with many systems.

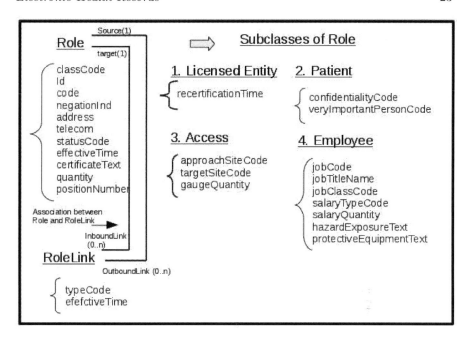

FIGURE 2.4: Role class [Source: [28]]

Furthermore, HL7 International is a standards organisation which engages volunteers (most without full-time commitments) in the development of standards specification. The volunteers have different levels of understanding and non-uniform lengths of participation in the process. The specifications are placed on ballots with required resolution of negative ballots. Therefore they are often prone to compromise, leading to ambiguity.

2.3.3 OpenEHR

OpenEHR provides technical specification for EHRs and EHR systems based on an object-oriented approach. Unlike HL7, which develops a standard for message exchanges in health informatics, the primary focus of the endeavour of the openEHR community is on electronic health records (EHR) and related systems. It puts forward a multilevel model with four major layers: (i) *a reference model*, (ii) *archetypes*, (iii) *templates*, and (iv) *template-generated artefacts*. Figure 2.6 shows the first three layers of openEHR.

A reference information model forms the basis of openEHR that defines the logical structure of EHRs and demographic data. The openEHR Foundation provides the specification of the reference model as a formal, logical definition of the information. Any healthcare provider storing EHR data in the openEHR system must obey this reference model. Demographic information is kept separate, so that a patient cannot be identified and the privacy of

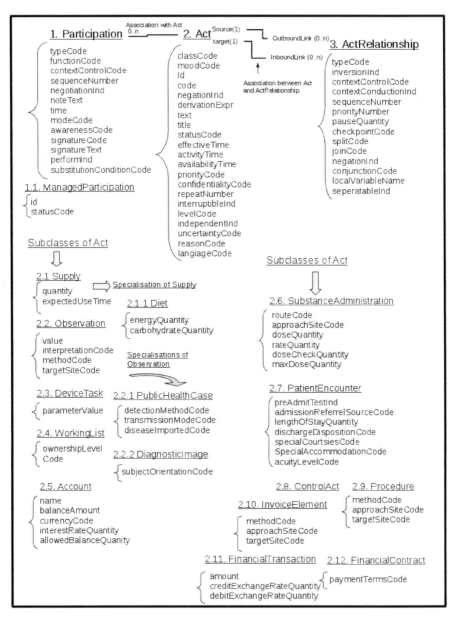

FIGURE 2.5: Participation class and its subclasses [Source: [28]]

the patient is maintained. However, the patient's information which is part of the health record (i.e., essential in this context) is stored. Versions of different data can also be stored. The following specifications are included in the

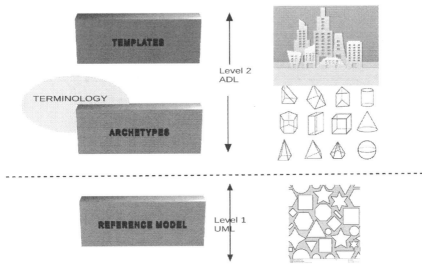

FIGURE 2.6: openEHR - multilevel modeling

reference model provided by the openEHR Foundation [20].

- **Task Planning Information Model—**
  Specifies the task lists and planned tasks.

- **EHR Information Model —**
  Specifies the information model of the EHR.

- **Demographic Information Model —**
  Specifies the openEHR demographics information model.

- **Common Information Model —**
  Specifies the information model containing common concepts, including the archetype-enabling LOCATABLE class, party references, audits and attestations, change control, and authored resources.

- **Data Structures Information Model —**
  This is the information model of data structures, including time-series data.

- **Data Types Information Model —**
  This is the information model of data types, including quantities, date/times, plain and coded text, time specification, multimedia and URIs.

- **Support Information Model** —
  The support model defines identifiers, assumed types, and terminology interface specification used in the other information models.

- **Integration Information Models** —
  This information model is used for representing legacy data in a free-form entry type for implementing integration solutions.

- **EHR Extract Information Model** —
  The information model is used for EHR Extract, which is a serialisation of content from an EHR.

Reference Model

Reference model includes a set of classes defining the generic structure of a patient health record. It also provides datatype definitions and assists in maintaining the versions of health data with appropriate specifications. The openEHR health record is arranged in a tree structure. The EHR for a single patient is placed at the root. Each EHR contains a unique, anonymous 'id', known as ehr_id. The 'id' is often associated with a real world identifier.

All of the patient data is contained in *compositions*. Compositions are organised into convenient groups for local use and these groups are placed in one or multiple *folders*. All recorded patient data are saved inside a composition. Every change in data creates a new version. Often, complex compositions are divided into *sections* for efficient management. A composition (or a section) contains a set of *entry* subclasses which carry all of the clinical payload. An *entry* can be *observation, evaluation, instruction, action,* or *admin entry*. The leaf nodes are actual datapoints, i.e., the *elements* which carry the values. Elements can have multiple occurrences. Elements are grouped into *clusters* which form the branch nodes inside an *entry*. The main openEHR classes along with a sample showing data objects of the classes are shown in Figures 2.7 and 2.8, respectively [1]. In general, UML is used for modeling at this level.

Archetypes

The level above the reference model consists of *archetypes*, which are computable models or patterns for capturing clinical information in the form of discrete clinical concepts. These archetypes are actually created as a library of data points and data groups which are independent of particular use and provide machine-readable specifications for how to store patient data using the openEHR reference model. Archetypes have been created for familiar components of a health record, such as blood pressure, body weight, and symptoms. For example, Figure 2.9 shows an archetype for blood pressure as available

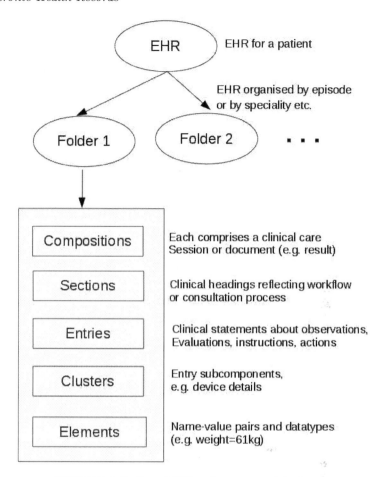

FIGURE 2.7: OpenEHR reference model classes

from the *Clinical Knowledge Manager* of openEHR Foundation. Archetypes are also created for representing clinical processes, and for recording and gathering information including patient history, physical examination, different courses of medicine, therapies, testing procedures, etc. They can also be used for recording outcomes of clinical assessments, such as diagnosis, genetic risk, allergy risk, etc. Additionally, there are also instruction archetypes for lab test request, referral, medication order, etc., and action archetypes to record the activities that result from an action. Archetypes are processed by archetype definition language (ADL). Additionally, they also include domain definition of information to add knowledge, XML-enabled lists, tables, time series data, etc.

The creation of a library of independent data groups removes the need for modeling the same group more than once. The other major advantage of using

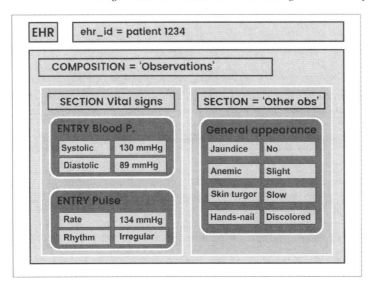

FIGURE 2.8: OpenEHR reference model classes — an example

archetypes is that these can be modeled even by clinical professionals who have no technological knowledge of the EHR systems. Thus, the archetypes are collaboratively authored, governed, and shared. It cannot be said that an archetype is complete and closed; rather, there is a continuous process for its further development, to maintain it and to keep it up to date. In fact, the motivation behind creating archetypes is the *maximal dataset* philosophy, i.e., capturing as many clinical perspectives as possible.

Multilingual archetypes have also been developed for several types of clinical information. Each archetype carries its own *terminology* to extend support for multiple languages.

Templates

At the top level, the archetypes are assembled into context-specific data sets, e.g., the data for a data entry form, a message for communication, or a document. These datasets created for a particular purpose are called *templates*. In a template, items can be made mandatory, unwanted items can be removed, default values can be set, and terminologies can be mapped to the data points. All openEHR systems are built with templates, which contain various archetypes that are relevant in the given context. Templates preserve the paths of archetype elements they use, even within variable depth structures. Templates are usually developed by implementers and are based on the local concepts related to the solution being built, but it is also possible to build standard templates for a region, or a country; e.g., a discharge sum-

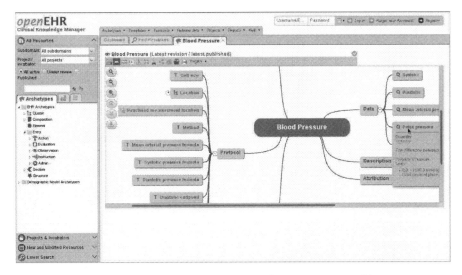

FIGURE 2.9: Archetype for blood pressure [Website: https://www.openehr.org/ckm/]

mary. The tools for template design and editing are provided by the openEHR Foundation.

The last level, closest to the user, are template-generated artefacts, such as application program interfaces. These artefacts are used by application developers. The openEHR Foundation provides the operational template specification.

Although, the archetypes are prepared by human beings and thus may contain errors, the openEHR Foundation endeavors to make the model safer for the EHR systems, and there is a continuous effort to make it interoperable with other popular standards. As of now, a total of 664 archetypes have been created, of which 515 are active and 149 have been deprecated or rejected. On the other hand, the total number of templates created so far is 78, and most of these templates either have been implemented as drafts or are in predraft or initial status. Details of openEHR archetypes and templates can be found in [21].

2.4   Adoption of EHR Standards

Adoption of EHR standards is being accelerated in different countries. In case of the American hospitals, doctors are subject to financial penalties under Medicare if EHRs are not utilised, In Europe, the EHR adoption rate is also increasing rapidly. For example, adoption of EHRs in France is almost close to that in USA [27]. The European, Middle Eastern, and African (EMEA) market is trailing behind that of the United States and is followed by the Asia Pacific market. Further discussion on the standards and Acts in different countries, particularly in the context of privacy of health data, is included in Chapter 8.

The BRIC countries, Brazil, Russia, China, and India, with their large population, are striving to adopt EHR standards which can be suitably used in their countries [22].

Brazil has framed interoperability standards for adoption at various levels of their national health system. The city of Sao Paulo adopted an open source EHR system called SIGA: the Saúde Health Information System. A national standard called Private Health Insurance and Plans Information Exchange Standard (TISS) has been established to support exchange of information among health providers and healthcare insurance companies. The standard will provide support for development of prototype software which will use an open EHR reference model to exchange TISS information.

An EHR system has been launched in Moscow, Russia, as part of the digital city program. The system facilitates booking of hospital visits and medical workers' shifts, online appointment services, management, and electronic prescribing based on cloud technology.

The Health Information Standards Professional Committee (HISPC) of the Ministry of Health (MOH) in China has prepared guidebooks describing standards and specifications for EHR and EMR systems which are to be adopted in China. The government has also taken the initiative to establish Regional Healthcare Information Networks (RHINs) for sharing data and clinical services among geographically dispersed communities.

With an objective to introduce a uniform standard for maintaining Electronic Health Records (EHRs) by healthcare providers in India, the Ministry of Health and Family Welfare of the Government of India introduced the Indian standard of EHR in 2013 [2]. Later, this standard was revised in consultation with the 'stakeholders' to incorporate contemporary developments, and a new document defining 'EHR standards 2016' has been released by the ministry [3].

The document provides an overview of all related standards. There is no mention of EHR-S. The standard does not define all attributes as mandatory, keeping in mind the Indian context. For every requirement in health informatics, the document clearly mentions which international standard is to be followed to implement EHR in India.

Patient identification is an issue in the Indian context as there is no single identification system to be followed for all purposes. Any patient-related attribute in this standard, alone or in combination with other attributes, can be used to identify a patient.

Patient Identification:

It is suggested in [3] that the unique 12-digit Aadhaar number provided to the Indian citizens by Unique Identification Authority of India, a government agency, should be considered as the preferable identifier whenever available. In the absence of this number, a local identifier, which is allotted within an institution or by a clinic or laboratory, may be treated as the patient identifier. Alternatively, a photo identity card number issued by the government may be used in conjunction with the local identifier. However, this may lead to a situation where different local identifiers along with photo identity card numbers are used for the same patient at different locations. Thus, a single person may become associated with different identities. In the absence of any direct methods for resolving such conflicts, the only possible way out is by devising smart algorithms for resolving these issues. An algorithm may use other parameters, such as name, address, date of birth, etc., to identify records belonging to the same person.

In addition to the standard specification for architectural and functional requirements, the standard defines the logical information reference model and structural composition, medical terminology and coding standards, data standards for image, multimedia, waveform and document, data exchange standards, etc. For example, it uses the ISO 13606 Health Informatics — Electronic Health Record Communication (Part 1 through 3) reference model and related specifications for the purposes of information model, architecture, and communication. On the other hand, openEHR Foundation Models Release 1.0.2 base model, reference model, and archetype model are used for the purpose of structural definition and composition. Optionally, this standard may also be used for service model, querying, and clinical decision support. Similarly, for data exchange, the following standards are specified: (i) event/message exchange is based on an application protocol for electronic data exchange in healthcare environments defined by ANSI/HL7 V2.8.2-2015 HL7 Standard Version 2.8.2, (ii) summary records exchange is based on ASTM/HL7 CCD Release 1, and (iii) EHR archetypes are based on ISO 13606-5:2010 Health informatics — Electronic Health Record Communication — Part 5: Interface Specification.

The document provides guidelines for implementation standards for hardware, software, networking, and connectivity. The document defines the data ownership of health records, and guidelines for privacy and security of health data.

The strongest point of this standard is that it has been prepared keeping in mind the Indian context. The main drawback of this standard is that it does not propose a data model. The minimum data set that it proposes does not seem to be complete.

2.5   Ontology-based Approaches

Section 2.3.1 has already discussed how *semantic interoperability* is necessary to interpret the information exchanged within the system and to relate that with the domain knowledge. Semantic interoperability of health informatics has been addressed by the standards, specifications, initiatives, and projects, such as ISO 13606 [1], openEHR [20], and HL7 [28]. In these standards and specifications, an EHR archetype is a formal specification of the data and their interrelationships, which logically persist within an EHR for documenting a particular clinical observation, evaluation, instruction, or action [12].

On the other hand, "ontology is the science of 'what is, of the kinds and structures of objects, properties, events, processes and relations' in every area of reality" [12]. Thus, ontologies can contribute to achieving semantic interoperability between EHRs by defining clinical terminologies for precise and sharable expressions, or by supporting transformations between different EHR standards. The difference between archetypes and ontologies are clarified by the openEHR Foundation: "An archetype for 'systemic arterial blood pressure measurement' is a model of what information should be captured for this kind of measurement — usually systolic and diastolic pressure, plus (optionally) patient state (position, exertion level) and instrument or other protocol information. In contrast, an ontology would describe in more or less detail what blood pressure is". [12]

Thus, ontologies can actually help to reduce the incompleteness in the EHR standards in terms of functionality by understanding the precise meaning of the underlying data. There have been several proposals for using the ontologies in this regard. González et al. [11] propose an interoperability framework that uses an ontology-based approach to support semantic interoperability among Electronic Health Records regardless of the EHR standard used.

Similarly, in [14], it is shown how two heterogeneous but similar drug administration models can be transformed into the ontology-based representation. This has been done through establishing the correspondences between clinical model data elements and ontology content patterns. Thus, ontologies can help to build more powerful and more interoperable information systems in healthcare.

2.5.1   Developing an Ontology

An ontology is developed through the following steps [19]:

- classes in the ontology are defined,

- classes are arranged in a subclass—superclass hierarchy,

- properties of the classes are defined. The value types, allowed values, number of values (cardinality) are defined for each property.

- instances of the classes are created, and

- values for instances are filled up.

Many ontologies are already available in electronic form and can be imported into an ontology-development environment. Thus, it is always wise to reuse the existing ontologies in order to save the time and effort of redoing the same task. There are some libraries of reusable ontologies on the web and these are also available in the literature. A survey of ontology libraries is available in [8], and it may be consulted by the readers to develop ontologies.

2.5.2   Ontologies for EHR

As pointed out earlier, obtaining a universal EHR for a patient is difficult for the various existing standards and specifications, and the heterogeneity of information systems. So the EHR needs to be developed within the framework of a federated information system. Hence, in order to share the knowledge between different EHR systems from the federation, a federated ontology is essential. Isabel Romàn proposes an ontology for a universal EHR [25]. The ontology is based on openEHR. Ontology files have been created, each of which corresponds to a reference model, and all are written in OWL ontology language (Web Ontology Language from W3C URL: https://www.w3.org/TR/owl2-syntax/) using Protege as editor.

Sil Sen et al. propose an ontology-driven approach to health data management for remote healthcare delivery. The main entities of the ontology are shown in Figure 2.10.

Figure 2.11 is an example of the classes instantiated during a patient's visit to a doctor. In this figure, types of entities are shown using straight lines, and relationships among different entities are shown using circles on dotted lines with arrows. Arrows point towards the parents, and where there are relationships, directions of the arrows indicate the directions of the relationships.

An example of inheritance of the classes is shown in Figure 2.12. Here the parent class is *history* with six subclasses.

A sample OWL file describing the inheritance of the *history class* is shown in Figure 2.13.

Every class is described with its data properties and object properties. When a property relates individuals to individuals, then it needs to be an object property, whereas if it relates individuals to literals, then it is used as a datatype property. Examples of data properties and object properties of a class *treatment episode* are given here. A *treatment episode* starts when a patient visits a clinic (or a doctor) with certain complaints. Thus, the entity is related to the entity *complaint* through the relationship *begins* and to the entity *visit* through the relationship *contains*. These relationships are shown in Figure 2.11. The corresponding OWL file describing the object properties of *treatment episode* is shown in Figure 2.14.

On the other hand, a *treatment episode* is described with several attributes like *start time, end time, type, status*, etc. The OWL file describing the data properties or attributes of *treatment episode* is shown in Figure 2.15.

2.5.3　Ontologies in Healthcare

Dang et al. [6] presents an ontological knowledge framework in a hospital domain. The domain includes the medical and administrative tasks in a hospital, hospital assets, medical insurances, patient records, drugs, and regulations. With this ontological framework, a user, who is either a doctor or a nurse or administrative staff, can (i) control and monitor the process flow that a patient will pass through, (ii) manage the patient's medical record and personal data, (iii) create new processes composed of tasks from a medical service repository, and (iv) maintain historical process data for future diagnosis.

Riaño et al. [24] developed an ontology for the care of chronically ill patients. The ontology does not aim to contain information about concrete patients (i.e., instances), but the clinical concepts, relationships, and constraints that are relevant to managing chronically ill patients. The clinical concepts include syndromes, diseases, social issues, signs and symptoms, problem assessments, and interventions. The ontology covers the domain knowledge related to nineteen diseases, such as anaemia, arthritis, chronic ischaemic heart disease, etc.

An ontology for primary healthcare in a Brazilian healthcare context has been proposed by Moraes et al. [16]. They defined the roles, legal terminologies, procedures, and relations which influence the primary healthcare domain. During the process, first the glossary of terms was decided to build the conceptualisation. Next, the concepts were integrated and the binary relations were defined. The ontology has been evaluated using *metric-based techniques* and *user evaluation*.

Larburu et al. observe that "pervasive healthcare systems apply information and communication technology to enable the usage of ubiquitous clinical data by authorized medical persons. However, quality of clinical data in these applications is, to a large extent, determined by the technological context of the patient". They find that the quality of clinical data may be degraded due to technological disruptions. Thus, an ontology is presented in [13] that specifies the relations among technological contexts, quality of clinical data (QoD), and patients' treatment. The framework consists of two parts: i) the technical domain ontology, which describes the technological knowledge and the relations between the technological contexts and the QoD relevant to clinical variables, and ii) the clinical domain ontology, which describes the clinical knowledge and the relations between the data quality relevant to treatment of the patients. Technological contexts include sensors, such as bio-harness sensors, or communication technologies, such as Bluetooth. On the other hand, clinical contexts include heart rate, etc.

Many other researchers have worked with ontologies, particularly in the healthcare domain. Ontologies are important for capturing the domain knowledge, and therefore are useful tools for developing the standards and specifications for healthcare, and also for integrating the heterogeneous systems to capture the diverse essence of them.

2.6   Chapter Notes

The chapter summarises different standards which are currently in use in different countries for storing and exchanging health information. First the definitions of EHR, EHR-S, and EMR are given. Next, some of the popular standards are discussed. The standards which have been discussed elaborately in this chapter include ISO/EN 13606, HL7, and open-EHR. One of the primary goals of defining these standards is not just achieving syntactic interoperability, but also semantic interoperaility. ISO/EN 13606 and open-EHR define a dual model architecture to separate information and knowledge in order to maintain semantic interoperability. While ISO/EN 13606 and open-EHR define how to store and retrieve data in an EHR-S, HL7 defines how messages are exchanged between two EHR systems.

Ontological approaches for representing health data are also discussed in this chapter. Examples are given to understand the basic design methodologies, and some earlier works have been summarised.

The basic objective of this chapter is to make the reader acquainted with different popular health informatics data models. It is not possible to include every detail in this book. For details, the readers may refer to the listed websites.

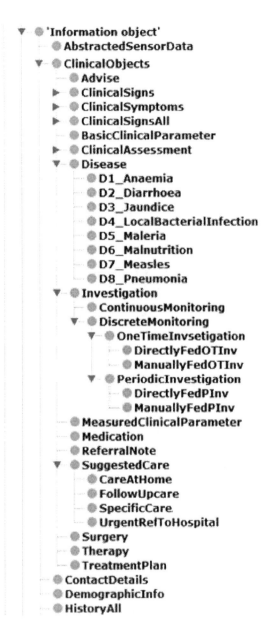

FIGURE 2.10: Hierarchy of different information objects in the ontology for health data of a remote health framework

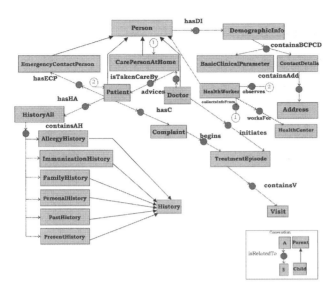

FIGURE 2.11: Entities involved during a patient's visit to a doctor

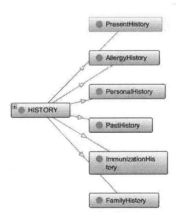

FIGURE 2.12: Inheritance of the patient's history class

```
<!-- http://www.semanticweb.org/aks/ontologies/2016/5/untitled-ontology-7#AllergyHistory -->
<owl:Class rdf:about="http://www.semanticweb.org/aks/ontologies/2016/5/untitled-ontology-7#AllergyHistory">
    <rdfs:subClassOf rdf:resource="&EHR_RM;HISTORY"/>
</owl:Class>
<!-- http://www.semanticweb.org/aks/ontologies/2016/5/untitled-ontology-7#ImmunizationHistory -->
<owl:Class rdf:about="http://www.semanticweb.org/aks/ontologies/2016/5/untitled-ontology-7#ImmunizationHistory">
    <rdfs:subClassOf rdf:resource="&EHR_RM;HISTORY"/>
</owl:Class>
<!-- http://www.semanticweb.org/aks/ontologies/2016/5/untitled-ontology-7#FamilyHistory -->
<owl:Class rdf:about="http://www.semanticweb.org/aks/ontologies/2016/5/untitled-ontology-7#FamilyHistory">
    <rdfs:subClassOf rdf:resource="&EHR_RM;HISTORY"/>
</owl:Class>
<!-- http://www.semanticweb.org/aks/ontologies/2016/5/untitled-ontology-7#PastHistory -->
<owl:Class rdf:about="http://www.semanticweb.org/aks/ontologies/2016/5/untitled-ontology-7#PastHistory">
    <rdfs:subClassOf rdf:resource="&EHR_RM;HISTORY"/>
</owl:Class>
<!-- http://www.semanticweb.org/aks/ontologies/2016/5/untitled-ontology-7#PersonalHistory -->
<owl:Class rdf:about="http://www.semanticweb.org/aks/ontologies/2016/5/untitled-ontology-7#PersonalHistory">
    <rdfs:subClassOf rdf:resource="&EHR_RM;HISTORY"/>
</owl:Class>
<!-- http://www.semanticweb.org/aks/ontologies/2016/5/untitled-ontology-7#PresentHistory -->
<owl:Class rdf:about="http://www.semanticweb.org/aks/ontologies/2016/5/untitled-ontology-7#PresentHistory">
    <rdfs:subClassOf rdf:resource="&EHR_RM;HISTORY"/>
</owl:Class>
```

FIGURE 2.13: OWL file describing the inheritance of the history class

```
<!-- http://www.semanticweb.org/aks/ontologies/2016/5/untitled-ontology-7#begins -->
<owl:ObjectProperty rdf:about="http://www.semanticweb.org/aks/ontologies/2016/5/untitled-ontology-7#begins">
    <rdfs:domain rdf:resource="http://www.semanticweb.org/aks/ontologies/2016/5/untitled-ontology-7#Complaint"/>
    <rdfs:range rdf:resource="http://www.semanticweb.org/aks/ontologies/2016/5/untitled-ontology-7#TreatmentEpisode"/>
    <owl:inverseOf rdf:resource="http://www.semanticweb.org/aks/ontologies/2016/5/untitled-ontology-7#initiatedFor"/>
</owl:ObjectProperty>
<!-- http://www.semanticweb.org/aks/ontologies/2016/5/untitled-ontology-7#containsV -->
<owl:ObjectProperty rdf:about="http://www.semanticweb.org/aks/ontologies/2016/5/untitled-ontology-7#containsV">
    <rdfs:domain rdf:resource="http://www.semanticweb.org/aks/ontologies/2016/5/untitled-ontology-7#TreatmentEpisode"/>
    <rdfs:range rdf:resource="http://www.semanticweb.org/aks/ontologies/2016/5/untitled-ontology-7#Visit"/>
</owl:ObjectProperty>
```

FIGURE 2.14: OWL file describing the object properties of the treatment episode class

```
<!-- http://www.semanticweb.org/aks/ontologies/2016/5/untitled-ontology-7#trtEpEndTimeStamp -->
<owl:DatatypeProperty rdf:about="http://www.semanticweb.org/aks/ontologies/2016/5/untitled-ontology-7#trtEpEndTimeStamp">
    <rdfs:domain rdf:resource="http://www.semanticweb.org/aks/ontologies/2016/5/untitled-ontology-7#TreatmentEpisode"/>
    <rdfs:range rdf:resource="&xsd;dateTimeStamp"/>
</owl:DatatypeProperty>
<!-- http://www.semanticweb.org/aks/ontologies/2016/5/untitled-ontology-7#trtEpId -->
<owl:DatatypeProperty rdf:about="http://www.semanticweb.org/aks/ontologies/2016/5/untitled-ontology-7#trtEpId">
    <rdfs:domain rdf:resource="http://www.semanticweb.org/aks/ontologies/2016/5/untitled-ontology-7#TreatmentEpisode"/>
    <rdfs:range rdf:resource="&xsd;string"/>
</owl:DatatypeProperty>
<!-- http://www.semanticweb.org/aks/ontologies/2016/5/untitled-ontology-7#trtEpNumber -->
<owl:DatatypeProperty rdf:about="http://www.semanticweb.org/aks/ontologies/2016/5/untitled-ontology-7#trtEpNumber">
    <rdfs:domain rdf:resource="http://www.semanticweb.org/aks/ontologies/2016/5/untitled-ontology-7#TreatmentEpisode"/>
    <rdfs:range rdf:resource="&xsd;integer"/>
</owl:DatatypeProperty>
<!-- http://www.semanticweb.org/aks/ontologies/2016/5/untitled-ontology-7#trtEpStartTimeStamp -->
<owl:DatatypeProperty rdf:about="http://www.semanticweb.org/aks/ontologies/2016/5/untitled-ontology-7#trtEpStartTimeStamp">
    <rdfs:domain rdf:resource="http://www.semanticweb.org/aks/ontologies/2016/5/untitled-ontology-7#TreatmentEpisode"/>
    <rdfs:range rdf:resource="&xsd;dateTimeStamp"/>
</owl:DatatypeProperty>
<!-- http://www.semanticweb.org/aks/ontologies/2016/5/untitled-ontology-7#trtEpStatus -->
<owl:DatatypeProperty rdf:about="http://www.semanticweb.org/aks/ontologies/2016/5/untitled-ontology-7#trtEpStatus">
    <rdfs:domain rdf:resource="http://www.semanticweb.org/aks/ontologies/2016/5/untitled-ontology-7#TreatmentEpisode"/>
    <rdfs:range rdf:resource="&xsd;string"/>
</owl:DatatypeProperty>
<!-- http://www.semanticweb.org/aks/ontologies/2016/5/untitled-ontology-7#trtEpType -->
<owl:DatatypeProperty rdf:about="http://www.semanticweb.org/aks/ontologies/2016/5/untitled-ontology-7#trtEpType">
    <rdfs:domain rdf:resource="http://www.semanticweb.org/aks/ontologies/2016/5/untitled-ontology-7#TreatmentEpisode"/>
    <rdfs:range rdf:resource="&xsd;string"/>
</owl:DatatypeProperty>
```

FIGURE 2.15: OWL file describing the data properties of the treatment episode class

References

[1] The ISO 13606 standard. Website: http://www.en13606.org/.

[2] Electronic health record standards for india. e-Health Division, Department of Health and Family Welfare, Government of India, August 2013.

[3] Electronic health record standards for india. e-Health Division, Department of Health and Family Welfare, Government of India, 2016.

[4] ISO/TC 215. Health informatics electronic health record definition, scope and context. Technical Report ISO/TR 20514:2005, International Organization of Standardization (ISO), 2005-10.

[5] ASTM standard practice for content and structure of the electronic health record (EHR). Website: http://www.astm.org/Standards/E1384.htm, January 2011.

[6] J. Dang, A. Hedayati, K. Hampel, and C. Toklu. An ontological knowledge framework for adaptive medical workflow. *Journal of biomedical informatics*, 41(5):829–836, 2008.

[7] A. Dogac, T. Namli, A. Okcan, G. Laleci, Y. Kabak, and M. Eichelberg. Key Issues of Technical Interoperability Solutions in eHealth and the RIDE Project. Technical report, Software R&D Center, Dept. of Computer Engg., Middle East Technical University, Ankara, 6531, 2007.

[8] Mathieu dAquin and Natalya F Noy. Where to publish and find ontologies? a survey of ontology libraries. *Web Semantics: Science, Services and Agents on the World Wide Web*, 11:96–111, 2012.

[9] S. H. El-Sappagh, S. El-Masri, A. M. Riad, and M. Elmogy. Electronic health record data model optimized for knowledge discovery. *IJCSI International Journal of Computer Science Issues*, 9(1):329–338, 2012.

[10] P. Garrett and J. Seidman. EMR vs. EHR what is the difference. Website: http://www.healthit.gov/buzz-blog/electronic-health-and-medical-records/emr-vs-ehr-difference/, January 2011.

[11] Carolina González, BG Blobel, and Diego M López. Ontology-based framework for electronic health records interoperability. *Studies in health technology and informatics*, 169:694–698, 2011.

[12] J. Grabenweger and G. Duftschmid. Ontologies and their application in electronic health records. *eHealth2008 Medical Informatics meets eHealth, Wien,* pages 29–30, 2008.

[13] N. Larburu, R. G. Bults, M. J. V. Sinderen, H. J. Hermens, et al. An ontology for telemedicine systems resiliency to technological context variations in pervasive healthcare. *IEEE journal of translational engineering in health and medicine,* 3:1–10, 2015.

[14] Catalina Martinez-Costa, MC Legaz-García, Stefan Schulz, and Jesualdo Tomás Fernández-Breis. Ontology-based infrastructure for a meaningful ehr representation and use. In *Biomedical and Health Informatics (BHI), 2014 IEEE-EMBS International Conference on,* pages 535–538. IEEE, 2014.

[15] C. N. Mead. Data interchange standards in healthcare IT – computable semantic interoperability: Now possible but still difficult. do we really need a better mousetrap? *Journal of Healthcare Information Management,* 20(1):71, 2006.

[16] E. Moraes, K. Brito, and S. Meira. Compophc: An ontology-based component for primary health care. In *2012 IEEE 13th International Conference on Information Reuse Integration (IRI),* pages 592–599, Aug 2012.

[17] P. Muoz, J. D. Trigo, I. Martnez, A. Muoz, J. Escayola, and J. Garca. The ISO/EN 13606 standard for the interoperable exchange of electronic health records. *Journal of Healthcare Engineering,* 2(1):1–24, 2011.

[18] C. Myer and J. Quinn. Hl7 overview. Website: `https://www.hl7.org/documentcenter/public_temp_05C9E67A-1C23-BA17-0C27F492CC603BE8/calendarofevents/himss/2008/presentations/HL7%20An%20Overview.pdf`, 2008.

[19] Natalya F. Noy and Deborah L. McCuinness. Ontology development 101: A guide to creating your first ontology. Website: `https://protege.stanford.edu/publications/ontology_development/ontology101-noy-mcguinness.html`.

[20] OpenEHR reference model. Website: `http://www.openehr.org/releases/RM/latest/docs/index`, 2017.

[21] OpenEHR Clinical Knowledge Manager. Website: `http://www.openehr.org/ckm/`.

[22] H. Parikh. Overview of EHR Systems in BRIC Nations. Website: `https://www.clinicalleader.com/doc/overview-of-ehr-systems-in-bric-nations-0001`, 2015.

[23] L. Pawola. The history of the electronic health record. Website: http://healthinformatics.uic.edu/the-history-of-the-electronic-health-record/, February 2011.

[24] David Riaño, Francis Real, Joan Albert López-Vallverdú, Fabio Campana, Sara Ercolani, Patrizia Mecocci, Roberta Annicchiarico, and Carlo Caltagirone. An ontology-based personalization of health-care knowledge to support clinical decisions for chronically ill patients. *Journal of biomedical informatics*, 45(3):429–446, 2012.

[25] Isabel Romn. Toward the universal electronic healthcare record (EHR) - an ontology for the EHR. Website: http://trajano.us.es/~isabel/EHR/.

[26] Health Level Seven. HL7 EHR system functional model: A major development towards consensus on electronic health record system functionality. Website: https://www.hl7.org/documentcenter/public/wg/ehr/EHR-SWhitePaper.pdf, 2004.

[27] C. P. Stone. A glimpse at EHR implementation around the world: The lessons the US can learn. Website: http://www.e-healthpolicy.org/docs/, May 2014.

[28] G. Tong. Introduction to HL7 version 3. Website: www.cas.mcmaster.ca/~yarmanmh/Recommended/v3Intro_e.pdf.

3

Big Data: From Hype to Action

CONTENTS

3.1   Introduction 43
3.2   What Is Big Data? 44
3.3   Big Data Properties 45
3.4   Why Is Big Data Important? 47
3.5   Big Data in the World 49
3.6   Big Data in Healthcare 50
    3.6.1   Is Health Data Big Data? 51
    3.6.2   Big Data: Healthcare Providers 52
3.7   Other Big Data Applications 54
    3.7.1   Banking and Securities 55
    3.7.2   Communications, Media, and Entertainment 55
    3.7.3   Manufacturing and Natural Resources 56
    3.7.4   Government 56
    3.7.5   Transportation 56
    3.7.6   Education 56
3.8   Securing Big Data 57
    3.8.1   Security Considerations 57
    3.8.2   Security Requirements 58
    3.8.3   Some Observations 59
3.9   Big Data Security Framework 59
3.10 Chapter Notes 61

3.1   Introduction

The term 'Big Data' is now heard everywhere. It has become a buzzword nowadays. Though it has become popular recently, the underlying challenges have existed for a long time. The rise of big data has increased the challenges in terms of privacy, security, and overall data management. Thus, problems also seem big with big data. However, it has also opened up the research area for big data analytics by exploring fundamental as well as evolving technologies. Specialised solutions are now coming up for specific big data applications.

3.2   What Is Big Data?

A perfect definition of big data may not be expressed in a single sentence. This is because of the fact that big data is usually viewed from different perspectives. Some say, "big represents the truest sense of the word *big*, that is, it is large, voluminous", others say, "it is big because it is increasing so rapidly!", and still others say, "no, it is big, because it represents various types".

Here we choose the following two observations regarding big data to arrive at its definition. As per Wikipedia [19]: "Big data is an all-encompassing term for any collection of data sets so large and complex that it becomes difficult to process them using traditional data processing applications."

As per Webopedia [17]: "Big data is a term, used to describe a massive volume of both structured and unstructured data that is so large that it's difficult to process using traditional database and software techniques. In most enterprise scenarios the data is too big or it moves too fast or it exceeds current processing capacity." Big data has the potential to help companies improve operations and make faster, more intelligent decisions.

Thus, the term big data may be defined as follows: Big data represents an exceedingly massive volume of rapidly changing structured, semi-structured, and unstructured data that is difficult to process using traditional data processing applications because of the complexity involved.

As we try to understand the real meaning of big data, we find that the term has been in use since the 1990s [13] [12]. Gartner [5] identified that data growth challenges and opportunities are three dimensional, and updated the definition as: 'Big Data is high-volume, high-velocity and/or high-variety information assets that demand cost-effective, innovative forms of information processing that enable enhanced insight, decision making, and process automation'. From then onwards these 3Vs were considered to be the characteristic pillars of big data. These are: Volume: the quantity and size of the generated and stored data. Variety: the types and features of the data. Velocity: the speed at which data is generated and processed to meet demands of various applications.

However, it was soon found that these 3Vs were not sufficient to fully describe the impact of big data. Thus the 3Vs have to be further expanded to accommodate other complementary characteristics of big data. Many more Vs have therefore been added to the original ones. Here we mention 8 Vs. All of them together represent the characteristics of big data: Veracity: the quality of the data. Variability: the same data value means different things in different contexts. Visualisation: a way of making data comprehensible. Volatility: Timeliness and validity of data. Value: knowledge gained from the data after analysis.

3.3 Big Data Properties

Let us start with the original three-dimensional model of the Vs.

Volume: The quantity of data generated from various applications is growing every day. As an example we may look into the following data: Google: 3.5 billion searches per day and 1.2 trillion searches per year worldwide [7].

The Internet in real time [18] [16] gives you the following statistics: By the time you finish reading this sentence, there will have been 219,000 new Facebook posts, 22,800 new Twitter tweets, and 7,000 apps downloaded. The amount of data uploaded to the Internet in a single second is a staggering 24,000 gigabytes.

Just see what happens in one Internet second: 54,907 Google searches, 7,252 Twitter tweets, 125,406 YouTube video views, and 2,501,018 emails sent [1].

The above statistics show the rate at which data is growing every second. Evidently there are varieties of data (text, pictures, and others) from innumerable different sources. Hence the quantity of the data itself is enormous. With the presence of social media (Twitter, blogs, Facebook, Instagram, to name a few), Internet search engines, and the large number of websites allowing online registrations and transactions, data is generated at a volume unlike anything seen before. And to top it all, several traditional applications are going digital, thereby generating large amounts of data.

Variety: Technically speaking, variety refers to different types of data formats. Commonly, data used to be stored as text, dat, and csv in sources such as filesystems, spreadsheets, and databases. This type of data usually has some fixed length and resides within a record or a file. This is what is called structured data, the kind that we were familiar with. Some types of data may not have a well-defined format, but the data fields may be represented using some kind of identifier or tag. This type of data may be called semi-structured data. As evident from the above, nowadays data is also generated in volumes from emails, message services, and other similar sources. Many such data may be combinations of text, audio, photos, or images and videos. In fact, the text itself may have several types of data (say, the date) embedded in it. We may not have any idea about the data type combination before handling it. Hence we may not know the expected format. This may be referred to as unstructured data. It is pretty obvious that these varieties of data formats would create problems in storing the data and analysing it as well.

Velocity: Generally velocity is defined to be the rate of change of position against time with respect to a reference frame. Hence, it seems perfectly fit for situations in which data is changing fast (every second, every minute, and so on) with respect to the earlier reference. It is as if new data is generated every second and the old data is not being deleted. So, we have a way of referring to the change the new data is bringing, with respect to the existing data.

Veracity: It seems reasonable that the accuracy of the data becomes a concern, with this huge amount of generated data. The user is concerned about the quality of the data. The user will expect the data to meet a given standard. Depending on the application and the sources of data generation, redundant data may be generated. Inaccuracy may also creep in. Adequate measures are to be taken so that the quality of the data remains.

Variability: Many times, the same data value may be generated in different contexts. This is particularly true for applications like email, blogging, messaging, etc. Some may use the word 'fine' to express positiveness, whereas in some other contexts it is an expression of frustration. Let us take the following example statements that serve to show the difference:
"Fine. Let us go." "Fine! Don't go, stay here." Here only the lexical meaning of *fine* will not bring out the actual semantics of the statements. We shall need to add the context in which the word is mentioned.

Visualisation: This large amount of data may sometimes look like haphazard data to a user. This is true for any non-trivial amount of data. There is always a need to present the data in such a manner that it is comprehensible. Hence it is important that the representation of the data be made understandable to one and all. The situation is the same where company reports are generated in such a way that a shareholder is able to understand even without going through the nuances. With big data, the problem of visualising the data arises from the fact that due to varieties of data, proper visualisation methods need to be chosen for each one, and the appropriate presentation must be made.

Volatility: Let us consider an example of patient monitoring. The ECG of an elderly patient is being monitored continuously The caregiver will take appropriate action whenever the ECG reading shows certain abnormality. Suppose the system is designed so that ECG data is coming hourly to the caregiver. The patient's readings may have deviated from the normal at 10:10 am, just after the regular hourly data had been posted at 10:00 am. This deviation will be noticed only at 11:00 am during the next hourly update. The action will be taken only after 11:00 am. It may be a very late action as the deviations could be fatal in nature. This shows that there is extreme importance of timeliness or freshness of the data. Big data volatility refers to how long data may be considered valid and how long it should be stored for further action. There is a need to determine at what point the data will no longer be relevant to the current analysis. The situation is akin to not using a medicine after its expiration date. The life span of the data may depend on the application, such that the data is usable. And since this data has high velocity, there is every chance of getting time-expired data.

Value: The question that is making its way into every mind is: What shall we do with so much data? We cannot just throw it away. We need to utilise it and gain experience. Substantial value can be found in big data. Applications may vary from optimising processes, understanding customers, and so on. As we find, traditional methods of exploring data may not be applicable to big data. So, new methodologies may be employed to analyse this huge amount of ever-changing data. Thereafter, we may gain some knowledge about the semantics of the data and use the knowledge in future. That is why everybody is keen to have big data analytics. With the other Vs and diverse properties of big data, value derived from big data will be more accurate, and hence, it will be used for precise prediction.

The properties of big data have made it special from day one. Because of these unusual properties, it has not been always possible to handle big data with the existing techniques and technologies. New technologies for storing big data, big data mining, and analytics have come into the market. People everywhere are busy trying their bit with big data - the buzzword of the decade.

However, generation of redundant data is a possibility in some applications. Hence, it may have to be *cleaned* before being used for its intended purpose.

3.4   Why Is Big Data Important?

Whether or not we are aware of it, big data has already enveloped our lives. Whatever we do, wherever we go, we are leaving our footprints everywhere in the digital world. We are also generating data even if we don't want to. Each of today's systems is generating more data than ever before. The software that operates such systems gathers data about what these systems are doing and the corresponding performances. Thus, this data is really too big, moves very fast, and does not always fit into the database strictures that we all are aware about. So, you have to find some alternative way to process this big data.

To give you some idea about the size of big data :

- 1000 Megabytes (MB) = 1 Gigabyte (GB)

- 1000 Gigabytes (GB) = 1 Terabyte (TB)

- 1000 Terabytes = 1 Petabyte (PB)

- 1000 Petabytes = 1 Exabyte (EB)

- 1000 Exabytes = 1 Zettabyte (ZB)

- 1000 Zettabytes = 1 Yottabyte (YB)

It seems that some more terminologies are going to be required soon. Such large bytes will require the storage of ever-growing files with varieties of data.

So, what does this big data look like? Big data can be anything ranging from chats in various social network sites, broadcast audio and video streams, online shopping and banking transactions, financial market data, to satellite imagery, GPS trails, and so on. The list is ever-growing. It is also interesting to note that the products and services that we deliver and consume generate a data flow back to the provider.

And here comes the most interesting fact! It is actually the ease with which we can use big data. We may not always have to own some specialised software for handling big data. Many times, you may not buy the software for yourself; the software required for processing is available in the cloud. Hence it may be shared among many users. It may be mentioned here that, according to Wikipedia [20] *"Cloud computing is an information technology paradigm that enables ubiquitous access to shared pools of configurable system resources and higher-level services that can be rapidly provisioned with minimal management effort, often over the Internet."*

The growth of big data is the culmination of years of market growth, trend analysis, and user demand, to name a few. However, the reasons for big data's having become so important all of a sudden may be attributed to the following facts:

- With continuous generation of huge data, it is easier to gain insight about the data regarding its sources and information. Depending on the requirement of the application, timely intervention is also possible.

- The power of data analytics became apparent, and businesses start taking advantage of the analytics, with a focus on bettering their performance.

- Because of the vast scope of developing technologies to cater to the requirements of big data, new directions are being envisaged.

- Handling different types of data formats all together opened new insights, and helped in gaining knowledge and developing insights from different perspectives.

Apart from the above, there also exist various micro-reasons that have contributed towards this unprecedented growth in big data.

3.5 Big Data in the World

The sources from which big data may be obtained vary, from Internet social media sites to real-time applications involving different sensors, and wireless sensor networks, and smart devices. So, it is pretty obvious that data obtained from these diverse sources will not always have the same format. And we already know that big data includes structured, semistructured and unstructured data. Also, since the range of applications is quite varied, sometimes processing of the data requires immediate attention. Many times, users employ mobile smart devices. Hence, data is obtained from mobile systems, too. It is apparent that data generated from static and mobile systems, including both infrastructured and adhoc systems, will be huge. The first concern is how to save and store these data. This is because of the fact that unless you save or store it, you are not able to process it.

It is unlikely that there will be large storage spaces in the organisations that deal with such large-volume, ever-changing data. Even if the storage is available, the overhead of its maintenance regarding regular backups, and safe and secured storage, will be huge. The organisations involved may not want to take this additional activity. So, the next best option for them will be to use some cloud storage. The motivating factors are more than one. These range from operational efficiency to strategic considerations. Ease of access with flexibility and data science and analytics capability are among the important ones. But it is not that easy for organizations to change their mindsets and jump to the new bandwagon of cloud.

Thus, cloud computing facilities get involved with big data. And once it is one of the likely candidates, organisations will always try to use this cloud facility. Cloud computing facilities may be used for a variety of purposes, like storage, computation, platform, and so on. This is all the more true because organisations may only have the traditional storage and database systems, which will not be sufficient for this new type of data. It is also a fact that organisations will try to maintain the status quo, until and unless and absolute necessity for change is felt by the authorities concerned.

Needless to say, this entire scenario, as described above, is already pushing the world towards a novel approach. The world is undergoing a change in its attitude, to accommodate this new feeling. In fact, the role of cloud in today's IT has grown significantly in response to changing market dynamics and emerging trends. However, the most challenging part for any application in big data is the collection of the intended data from varied sources. The data may actually be scattered at places and difficult to put together in one place for effective analysis. This is because the world was not ready until recently to realise the power of this enormous amount of data lying strewn all over the place. But now that the potential is being realised, everybody is scurrying to have all the data together for better utilisation.

The upfront challenge with big data is its unstructured nature. This makes it difficult to categorise, model, and map the data when it is generated or captured and stored. Since the data normally comes from external sources, it gets hard to confirm its accuracy. Therefore, organisations have to identify what information is of value for their business. Capturing all the information available may unnecessarily waste time and resources, and put them at risk, thereby adding little or no value to the business [10].

Big data meeting the cloud and mobile worlds is a game-changer for businesses of all sizes.

3.6   Big Data in Healthcare

The healthcare sector has access to huge amount of data. But even today, not all data is in an electronic format, and hence, it is not utilised properly. However, the trend is towards converting all healthcare data into an electronic format. Then it will be easier for doctors to treat patients, since all information (past and present) regarding a patient would be there at the click of a mouse. Along with this, the important supplement is the implementation of proper data analysis strategies and tools, without which this huge potential will remain under utilised.

There are different sources and types of health data. These data are stored in different storehouses and accessed and retrieved. The variation in the types of data prove that it is indeed a complex and tough task to store such data and retrieve it accordingly. The analysis to be performed and the inferences to be drawn will again lead the system towards the next phase. This next phase may be some business decision or inputs for research on some specific field or even a future treatment plan.

Big data in healthcare will be utilised for providing cures for diseases, predicting epidemics, and improving quality of life. Such prediction will help doctors avoid preventable deaths [11].

3.6.1 Is Health Data Big Data?

A general terminology is indicated in [9], whose extent is bounded by health-related information and corresponding data values. In reality, health data is health related information about a person; in particular, a patient.

Let us consider a scenario where a patient visits any hospital or health clinic for the first time. The patient will be involved in a series of activities, may be beginning with filling in a registration form mentioning his details, such as, name, address, phone number, and age, to start with. This data will be accompanied by healthcare professionals taking over for measuring height, weight, blood pressure, and pulse rate, to name a few. These initial activities may not involve the doctor. The healthcare professional may also indicate general symptoms that the patient refers to as reasons for visiting the hospital. After being examined by the doctor, the patient may be asked to take a few more diagnostic tests, such as different types of blood tests, ECG, USG, and so on. So the data about the patient now comprises all such information that includes text, images, and images embedded with text. In extreme cases, this may include videography, such as angiography.

Health data sources are numerous, and include Wireless Body Area Networks (WBANs). Patients with WBAN can be monitored from remote locations. A plethora of technologies including wireless technologies will be necessary to develop and maintain such a large healthcare system. Different types of wearable devices including sport fitness devices are also part of this. Data from diverse sources also include real-time monitoring data, data of chronic diseases, complaints and symptoms of the patients, and early diagnostics, to name a few. All of these form the Internet of Things (IoT) system for healthcare.

The doctor will be able to arrive at some diagnosis (with all the above-mentioned technological aids), prescribe medicines, and may ask to have a follow-up checkup sometime soon. Thus, the health data of the patient increases day by day. And we are not talking about only one patient here. There are a number of hospitals with different medical departments and with numerous patients visiting these departments daily. All this data is in digital format and forms the Electronic Health Record (EHR). Therefore, the EHR can be considered to be a digital version of a patients paper chart. EHRs are real-time, patient-centred records. They are able to provide information available not only instantly but also securely to authorised users.

The data is thus growing in leaps and bounds, and it involves data in various formats. Apart from this, the hospitals will have in-house patients who are being regularly monitored. Some of these patients may have various wearable sensor devices required for continuous monitoring. Sensor devices will generate huge data in no time.

An EHR contains all medical and treatment histories of a patient. It contains laboratory test results, and radiology images, among other things. Thus, the different types of data in an EHR are huge, ever growing, valuable. The properties of big data are thus evident in these EHRs. This data has to be stored and analysed in such a way that it generates information that will be helpful in future. This is the pointer towards big data analytics.

It is quite apparent that healthcare is overflowing with data accumulated from various sources [3]. Analysis of such different types of voluminous data will bring out its essence with important and precise information. This can enhance clinical decision support. Data consumers are also quite inquisitive and want to gain knowledge. Their demand is for useful information, so that they can facilitate their healthcare decisions on their own. However, data has to be used correctly to get better understanding of healthcare choices.

On the other hand, when captured by doctors, this critical information will be used to improve decision making and insights into disease states. For example, using sophisticated computerised decision support that incorporates knowledge of the patient, a pharmacist may be able to detect potentially dangerous drug interactions as well. Timely alert-generation and other actions may then take place.

3.6.2   Big Data: Healthcare Providers

The world's population is not only increasing, but also living longer. With advancement in medical technology and treatments, models of treatment delivery are also rapidly changing. And one of the reasons behind this is the analysis of different data that the healthcare industry is now generating and storing. The healthcare professionals now want to know as much about a patient as possible, so that proper care may be taken as early as possible, in the correct direction. In a nutshell, the potential of healthcare analytics lies in reducing healthcare costs, predicting outbreaks of epidemic diseases, and avoiding preventable diseases, among other things. This would definitely enhance quality of life.

Nowadays the younger generation is particularly hooked to smart devices. So, why not start with apps to offer them better healthcare for the future? There are different smart apps that start with taking note of the number of steps you take to the calories you are taking in, to the calories you need, to reminding you of your daily medicines, to whatever. There are *Fitbit* [2], *Samsung Gear Fit* [15], and so on, which will take your data and analyse it so that you track yourself on all fronts where you want to be healthier.

As mentioned in 3.6.1, we see that the time is not so far off when the doctor will be able to get all the details of the patient as soon as the patient visits the doctor with new complaints. However, this means access to an ever-growing database of health records by the doctors and other medical professionals. The other perspective is that this data is not in isolation but will be analysed and compared with millions of other data. Sophisticated modeling of this analysis will give rise to patterns that can be predicted. Hence, the patient will get to have a directed, individualised treatment.

There are still other ways that this enormous data will be utilised. Let us take the example of drug companies. They will require information regarding certain diseases or the sale of certain drugs, maybe during some particular time interval, and so on. They will never need the identities of the patients but may require the count as to how many prescriptions are handed out for some particular drugs. They may also need the demographic information of the patients, so as to find out the medicine requirements in a certain geographic region. Another perspective is from the drug research organisations. They will use all such information and analyse patterns of occurrences of disease, patterns of drug usage, etc., to discover new drugs, treatments, or medical insights. Healthcare therefore requires more future-oriented tools of machine learning, predictive analysis, and graph analytics.

Data from seemingly simple scenarios is actually helping healthcare professionals gain insight. For example, if a hospital has the records of admissions over the past few years, then the admission rate will be able to speak for itself. This data may be analysed to find the minimum and maximum rate during time of the day, time of the year, and hence, the requirements of staff can be predicted and the hospital will be ready beforehand. Electronic Health Records (EHRs) guarantee a patient's health-related information at one go. It enables doctors to go through the history data as well and prescribe new medicines, and tests. No data will be overwritten or replicated. Implementation of EHRs has indeed increased savings in healthcare.

With the help of the Clinical Decision Support (CDS) system and the patient health information, medical practitioners will be able to gain insight and then arrive at prescriptive decisions. This may well be used for generating health alarms. Statutory warnings may be generated and patients can be made aware of certain situations. CDSs may be used an aid that can guide healthcare providers at remote places, to provide necessary advice to the patient before a medical professional steps in.

Predictive analytics is, of course, one of the most interesting business-intelligence trends in healthcare. Its primary aim is to help doctors make an improved big-data informed decision within seconds. The secondary aim should be predicting patients which are at risk for diabetes or hypertension, and so on. Thus, additional checkups and other screening or diagnostic tests may be performed on them regularly.

Another interesting outcome may be to use big data analytics to find a cure for certain so-called incurable diseases. For a particular disease, the patient information, complete with demographics and usage pattern of medicines, treatment, and schedule, along with success rate, is now available, thanks to big data. Why not use such analytics to find out the success rate of reusing this pattern on patients with similar demographics and health records? Who knows, the day may not be far off when we shall have cure in sight for those so-called incurable diseases.

Obviously, it is always easier said than done! The issue of privacy regarding patients will come up here. Though actual patient identification may not be required, the probability of the patient being identified is there, since all other information, including demographics, will also be used. Also, an institution may not be eager to share such information with others, citing their patient confidentiality clause.

3.7 Other Big Data Applications

Big data has already taken the world by storm. Till now, people were wondering what to do and how to handle this data. Hence, it remained more or less unused. But people are intelligent enough to recognise the latent talent in big data. Thus, big data is now being considered as having great value. This is because of the power lying hidden in big data analytics, as the industries have now come to realise.

Distribution of different characteristics of big data over different industries and in government is also available in various studies. Here we focus on some of the applications of big data that are driving the industries of today [4] [8]. These are mentioned in [4].

3.7.1 Banking and Securities

The main challenges that these industries face are warnings regarding securities fraud, financial data analytics, detection of fraud in credit/debit cards, trade visibility and market acceptance, customer data handling and management, social analytics for numerous purposes, IT operations analytics, and IT policy compliance analytics, among others. It seems that everybody in the financial market, including the U.S. Securities and Exchange Commission, traders, banks, and hedge funds, are using big data analytics. The analytics are being used for purposes suitable to the respective parties, such as, predictive analytics, pre-trade decision support analytics, and so on. Risk analytics is also involved in a major role with demand enterprise risk management, *know your customer*, and fraud mitigation. Big data providers specific to this industry include 1010data, Panopticon Software, Streambase Systems, Nice Actimize, and Quartet FS.

3.7.2 Communications, Media, and Entertainment

This is a very sensitive industry, with respect to the expectations and demands of consumers. They expect rich on-demand media in all formats and in all devices, irrespective of where the user or the source of the media is located. So, the challenges are many, and include:

1. Consumer requirements collection and analysis
2. Leveraging mobile and social media content
3. Understanding patterns of usage
4. Understanding requirement regarding content delivery, real-time necessity

Analytics may drive the industries to maintain individual user profiles for better marketing. This will include content creation and recommendation for different target audiences, and measuring content performance as well. As an example, we can take Spotify, an on-demand music service. It collects data from its worldwide users, and uses Hadoop big data analytics to provide informed recommendations to individual users. Big data providers in this industry include Infochimps, Splunk, Pervasive Software, and Visible Measures.

3.7.3 Manufacturing and Natural Resources

There has been an increasing demand for natural resources like oil, agricultural products, minerals, gas, and metals for the ever-growing world population. Information regarding the occurrences of natural oil, gas, and metal resources, and the suitability of land for agricultural purposes, include geographical, climate, and temporal data. This has led to big data analytics being used for predictive modeling. The analytics may also be used for seismic interpretation.

Manufacturing industries for their part, are already generating huge data. But this is still untapped. The world is now facing global warming challenges, go-green challenges, and quality production challenges, among others. The analysis of this data will be helpful for energy management on the one hand, as well market profit trends, and improvements in quality products, on the other.

3.7.4 Government

The biggest challenge that any government faces is integration and interoperability among different government departments, and affiliated organisations. Use of medical information may aid in social services, such as, services that target diseases or help people with special needs. In an agricultural country like India, descriptive land records analytics along with climatic information will help in the prediction of crop production. Above all, different types of data from varied sources may be analysed for the security of the country.

3.7.5 Transportation

Due to the increase in location-aware softwares and mobile applications, huge data is generated every few seconds. Crowd sensing has already become a very effective way of data collection. However, there does not seem to be adequate understanding of the nature of the data, and so it is under utilised. Both government and private agencies will benefit from this data if there is a proper model for utilization. It can then be used for traffic control and management, logistics for travel, route planning, and congestion avoidance, to name a few. This will lead to the development of intelligent transportation systems.

3.7.6 Education

This sector has large and varied data that individual institutions as well as other agencies can utilise. Any educational institution can provide an online learning management system that will provide it with data about students. This data may help in developing similar products by studying trends. Agencies may similarly use data in predicting the future requirements in number and variety of education trends. Overall, student behavioural classification, aspirations, performance, and job analysis will help in developing the system further.

Apart from the ones mentioned above, applications in other industries are also found.

3.8   Securing Big Data

This new era of big data is dynamic in nature. It is relentlessly producing a large amount of data. The interesting and important part related to this production is that this data is giving us greater insights into exciting new research areas and leading us to make better business decisions. Of course, in many ways, this is indeed valuable for customers. Organisations therefore must be able to handle data efficiently, timely, and securely, because often this data will include sensitive information [6].

It is only natural that every business wants to derive business intelligence (BI) from this data. Obviously, it is not an easy task to analyse this massive data and find out the key information. This is not the only task. The other important task, which is sometimes overlooked, is the task of ensuring that the data is not leaked or revealed to unwanted persons.

Thus, big data really brings with itself a number of security issues. The security issues are also big because of the nature of the data. The big security problem of big data is commonly attributed to the property of *variety*. This is because each type of data will have its own security problem depending on its nature. For example, the threat to text data will be different in nature from the threat to image data. Thus, the protection to be provided will also vary with the nature of data; that is, its variety.

3.8.1   Security Considerations

Managing big data security is really a big task. Hence, security has to be provided from different perspectives. These include *Infrastructure Security and Integrity, Data Privacy,* and *Integrity and Reactive Security, Identity and Access Management.* However, the rigor of security depends on the application requirement. So, management may also have to decide on the perspective of security or privacy it has to emphasise.

There are lots of expectations from big data. These expectations are from all categories of stakeholders: sources of big data, designers and developers of big data applications, designers of big data storage facilities, users, and so on. All business leaders are into big data now. But to actually reap the benefits of big data, the data needs to be not only properly analysed but also correctly inferred. This is what can be called big data analytics. Though the rewards of big data are great, there are some risks involving security.

As already mentioned above, there are numerous sources from which big data is generated. Developers of the application must have enough knowledge to identify the proper information to be extracted from data, since all fields in a data item may not be required. The sources of data also need proper validation. It may so happen that for some applications, data from a source has to traverse a long path, hopping from one intermediate node to another. This entire path has to be taken care of. The network node at which data will be encrypted and decrypted has to be identified, since encrypted data may take more time to be saved and retrieved. Appropriate metadata need to be kept for encrypted data.

User access control policies have to be well planned to thwart unauthorised access. There has to be enough surveillance to detect any attack or even the possibility of an attack. For example, if it is detected that a fraudulent transaction on a credit card is on the way, it has to be stopped midway before it gets completed.

Sometimes data (particularly, video or image) has to be compressed. During this transformation, sensitive data must not be exposed. Sometimes, a few fields of a data item may remain null. Developers have to be cautious so that during computation, sensitive data and null values are properly used.

Health data in EHR must be handled according to the laws of the land. Location-based services require user location, and so this may be exposed globally. Data in social media must be shared so as to carefully consider all consequences.

3.8.2   Security Requirements

It is apparent that generally, authentication, authorisation, cryptography, and integrity checking may be mandatory for all applications. Public key cryptography and Symmetric key cryptography are the widely used methods for providing security. The first type uses two different keys: public and private, while the second type uses only one key. Application requirements may be somewhat more specific and need stringent security measures other than the default ones. The requirements for these features are an appropriate storage and retrieval facility, and a proper security level from the perspective of the application.

Users would require an interface that offers easy navigation, so that they can be easily authenticated and authorised. Privacy is sometimes a requirement, that should be provided, too. The responsibility of seamless distribution or generation of different keys required for security purposes must be on servers or devices, or some other similar entities.

The primary requirement for data is confidentiality and integrity. Sensitivity of data is also an issue, particularly in some applications. All the V's of big data have to be treated the way they demand. A significant feature may be the relevance of the data, since a large amount of data will be generated. And it is always desired that the system be available whenever the user wants it.

3.8.3   Some Observations

With big data in our hands, known use cases may have to be redefined to fit the criteria. Since data may be sensitive, timely detection of anomalous retrieval is very necessary. Data anonymisation is also required for privacy purposes. What is to be done is that a balance involving these three **Network-centric**, **Access Control-centric** and **Data-centric** approaches are required to obtain a security solution for big data.

3.9   Big Data Security Framework

Security provisioning for big data systems will require appropriate security architecture. The architectural model will identify the logical building blocks and their interrelationships. A big data security framework is described below. The core components of the framework are:

1. Data Management: The most important task in this area is data classification. After determining all distinct data fields, corresponding threats or security breaches have to be identified. The users associated with these data fields are also to be identified. This is because of the fact that different attributes of a data item may be provided by different sources. For example, in the case of health data, pathological reports will be provided by the laboratories, whereas diagnosis and thereby the name of the disease will be provided by the medical practitioner.

    It is also important to find whether the data will be useful to others in the system, or anyone else, since these users may be a source of malicious activities. With all such information, it may be possible to have an idea of an attack that may take place, or sometimes to identify the categories of attacks. Thereafter, the damage that may be done by these attacks can be evaluated and a proper mitigation plan devised.

Since big data has both structured and unstructured data, the way of handling sensitive data will vary. While there may be cell-level identification in the case of structured data, for unstructured data, this may have to depend on schema identification and conditional search routines, or specific use-cases scenarios.

Data tagging will be helpful in identifying all different sources of data as well their exit points. This will provide the boundaries within which a particular data item will work. This may provide flexibility to designers in modeling and managing the data accordingly.

2. Identity and Access Management: Generally, centrally managed access control policies are implemented in big data systems. However, a word of advice may be to link policy to data and not access methods. This means that type and sensitivity of data may dictate policy. The system that handles sensitive data may require an access policy dependent on user as well as data attributes, which is different from a system that deals with not-so-sensitive data. The access policy of the system that does not deal with sensitive data may simply be based on user role in the system.
Whatever the access policy may be, real-time monitoring should be done in any system. The usage pattern of a user may be monitored, and too-frequent access may raise the suspicion level. If there are repeated failed attempts to log into an account, that should also be noted and action taken.
A system that does not generally deal with sensitive data may use special tags to identify sensitive data, in case the need arises. This would take special care of the sensitive data so that it is not unduly accessed.

3. Data Protection and Privacy: Many applications provide application-level cryptographic protection. However, if the requirement is more stringent, encryption may be provided at the level of data field, too. But measures have to be taken to identify only those data fields that need protection, otherwise it would unnecessarily complicate the system.
Besides this, there can be full disk encryption. But this would also unnecessarily be a burden. Data masking is another well-known

technique of hiding real or actual data during the development process. Any of these or combinations of them can be used for protecting data.

4. Network Security: Security-enabled protocols are now available for different layers in the network architecture. **Transport layer Security (TLS)** is responsible for authentication and privacy of communications. Besides TLS, LDAP, SSL are also there. Packet-level encryption may also be used.

   Typically, *zoning* is also used. Zoning is aimed at segmenting similar information technology assets into logical groupings for selectively allowing access to data. To implement the concept of *zoning*, first, different points in a cluster or region or network have to be identified. Then, measures have to be taken to restrict users beyond those points. User A may go to a certain point X, whereas some other user B may be allowed to go to point Y in the network. Use of firewalls is also an age-old but widely practiced solution.

5. Infrastructure Security and Integrity: A system always generates logs of events. The next step would be to protect these logs from being tampered with. Apart from this, file level integrity checking should also be made mandatory. Monitoring of big data clusters may be done by audit logging technologies (such as Apache Oozie).

The big data security framework emphasises understanding every aspects of the data in order to find the sensitive data among the huge *big* data. This is required because since only sensitive data needs special treatment. Once sensitive data is identified, the next step is to develop a solution for securing the data and implementing the solution. This would finally secure the data. However, the need for monitoring never ends. Hence, monitoring would go on with an aim to control access oo the data. This gives rise to default mitigation as well as *on-the-fly* mitigation strategies. Analysis and mitigation now become a continuous cycle [14].

3.10 Chapter Notes

This chapter focuses on Big Data in a BIG way. Starting with the definition, properties, the hype, and the application areas, the chapter has dealt with all these aspects of big data. The healthcare application is dealt with specially, since this book is going to be about healthcare and analytics.

References

[1] DailyMail. Internethappenings. http://www.internetlivestats.com/one-second/#traffic_band, 2017.

[2] Eric and James. Fitbit Versa. https://www.fitbit.com/home, 2018.

[3] Helen Figge. Harnessing Data for Healthy Outcomes. https://www.uspharmacist.com/article/harnessing-data-for-healthy-outcomes, 2014.

[4] Maryanne Gaitho. How Applications of Big Data Drive Industries. https://www.simplilearn.com/big-data-applications-in-industries-article, 2017.

[5] Gartner. GARTNER IT GLOSSARY : BIG DATA. In *Gartner IT Glossary: What is Big Data?* 2013.

[6] Gemalto. Big Data Security Solutions. https://safenet.gemalto.com/data-encryption/big-data-security-solutions/, 2016.

[7] Google. Googlesearchstatistics. http://www.internetlivestats.com/, 2017.

[8] Intellipat. 7 Big Data Examples Application of Big Data in Real Life. https://intellipaat.com/blog/7-big-data-examples-application-of-big-data-in-real-life/, 2017.

[9] S. M. Riazul Islam, Daehan Kwak, and Md. Humaun Kabir. The Internet of things for healthcare: A Comprehensive Survey. *IEEE Access*, 3:678–708, 2015.

[10] Guillermo Lafuente. Big Data Security – Challenges & Solutions. https://www.mwrinfosecurity.com/our-thinking/big-data-security-challenges-and-solutions/, 2014.

[11] Mona Lebled. 9 Examples of Big Data Analytics in Healthcare That Can Save People. https://www.datapine.com/blog/big-data-examples-in-healthcare/, 2017.

[12] Steve Lohr. The Origins of Big Data: An Etymological Detective Story. *New York Times*, 2013.

[13] John R. Mashey. Big Data ... and the Next Wave of InfraStress. static.usenix.org/event/usenix99/invited_talks/mashey.pdf, 1998.

[14] Aviv Ron, Alexandra-Shulman-Peleg, and Anton Puzanov. Analysis and Mitigation of NoSQL Injections. https://www.infoq.com/articles/nosql-injections-analysis, 2017.

[15] Samsung. Gearfit2. http://www.samsung.com/global/galaxy/gearfit2/, 2018.

[16] Twitter. New Tweets per second record, and how! https://blog.twitter.com/engineering/en_us/a/2013/new-tweets-per-second-record-and-how.html, 2013.

[17] Webopedia. Big Data. http://www.webopedia.com/TERM/B/big_data.html, 2017.

[18] WebPage. Real-Time-Internet. https://www.webpagefx.com/internet-real-time, 2017.

[19] Wikipedia. Bigdata. https://en.wikipedia.org/wiki/Big-data, 2017.

[20] Wikipedia. Cloud Computing. https://en.wikipedia.org/wiki/Cloudcomputing, 2018.

4

Acquisition of Big Health Data

CONTENTS

4.1 Introduction 65
4.2 Wireless Body Area Network 66
    4.2.1 BAN Design Aspects 68
    4.2.2 WBAN Sensors 70
    4.2.3 Technologies for WBAN 70
        4.2.3.1 Bluetooth and Bluetooth LE 70
        4.2.3.2 ZigBee and WLAN 71
        4.2.3.3 WBAN standard 71
    4.2.4 Network Layer 73
    4.2.5 Inter-WBAN Interference 74
4.3 Crowdsourcing 76
4.4 Social Network 79
4.5 Chapter Notes 83

4.1 Introduction

The healthcare sector is buzzing with data. It can be easily perceived that this data belongs to various types or categories and is therefore expressed in various different formats.Thus health data has earned itself the tag of *Big Health Data*. Obviously, the pertinent questions crop up - how is this data generated and how can this data be acquired and retained or stored thereafter.

This chapter throws light on acquisition of Big Health Data. Acquisition methodology and method thereof will be different for different types of healthcare application. For example, application like remote patient monitoring will require patients to have access to health sensors so that data from sensor nodes be continuously fed into the application. The most suitable way is to have sensors attached to or implanted in the body of patients. Wireless Body Area Network (WBAN or BAN) is the implementation of this concept. Similarly, Social media platforms (Social Networks) are found to be suitable for applications that require spreading awareness and / or acquiring information about certain health conditions.

4.2 Wireless Body Area Network

A wireless body area network (WBAN or BAN) comprises small, intelligent sensors attached to the body or implanted in the body. They set up wireless communication links among themselves, as shown in Figure 4.1. These devices are capable of monitoring health continuously and they can also provide real-time health data to the user, medical personnel or to any other entity. It may be possible to do these tasks manually, but recording the measurements for a longer period of time or recording them without the intervention of a medical practitioner is not possible without deploying a WBAN.

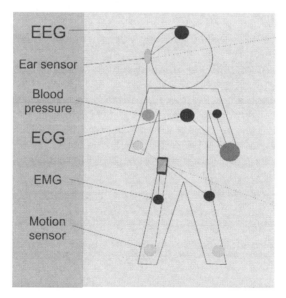

FIGURE 4.1: Sensor on human body

A WBAN comprises sensors and actuators. Sensors measure certain parameters of a human body. For example, sensors may gather electrocardiogram (ECG) data, measure temperature of the body, or the number of heartbeats. Depending on the data measured by the sensors, actuators take appropriate actions. Suppose that an actuator is equipped with a built-in reservoir and pump. Depending on the glucose level measured by a sensor placed on a patient's body, the actuator may push the appropriate dose of insulin. In a WBAN, the sensors send the data to a sink which is typically a PDA or a smart phone.

Protocols and algorithms of wireless sensor networks and wireless ad hoc networks may also be applied for communication between the sensor devices on, in, and around the body. But WBAN has characteristics which make it very difficult for exisiting protocols and algorithms of WSN or ad hoc networks to be applied on a WBAN. Unlike a wireless sensor network, there are no redundant nodes in a WBAN, and thus, all nodes in a WBAN are equally important. Transmission power for these nodes must be maintained very low. This helps in minimising interference. High power also raises the temeprature of body tissues, and absorption of electromagnetic transmission involve serious health concerns. The devices in a human body can be moving. So, WBAN must be able to cope with frequent changes in network topology. High reliablity and low latency are also required for on-time delivery of critical data. The differences between characteristics of WBAN and that of WSN are concisely available in [24].

While WSN cover areas measured in metres or kilometres, length of WBAN networks is limited by the length of a human body. WSN involves a large number of nodes so that the entire area can be covered well. But WBAN comprises very small number of nodes. Accuracy of a WSN is obtained by deploying a large number of redundant nodes while accuracy of a WBAN is achieved by precsion of the nodes themselves. WSN toplogy may be fairly fixed but WBAN topology has to be dynamic due to relative movement of body parts. WSN sensor nodes need not be biocompatible but WBAN sensor nodes must be biocompatible as they are implanted or are in contact with body tissues. All WSN applications do not need to be secured but WBAN applications have to secured as they deal with patient data. In a WSN, lots of redundant nodes are present to compensate for data loss but QoS and data delivery must be ensured in WBANs. In WBAN, low power technology has to be used but this is not mandatory for all WSN applications.

WBAN is supposed to support a host of applications, spanning the medical field, entertainment, gaming, and ambient intelligence areas. Vital sign monitoring and automatic drug delivery are two common applications in the medical field. This panorama of applications creates a wide variety of technical requirements that have to support very different performance metrics. To support such diverse applications, protocols and architectures must be adaptive and flexible. In WBAN, the following communication protocols are primarily used: IEEE 802.15.4 [19], IEEE 802.15.6 [20], and Bluetooth Low Energy [18].

There are three conceptual tiers in a typical WBAN architecture, as shown in Figure 4.2. Tier 1 corresponds to Intra-WBANs. In this tier, sensor nodes on the body or implanted in the body transmit the sensed data to the base station or the coordinator. Tier 2 corresponds to Inter-WBANs. In this tier, coordinators transmit the received data to the sink(s). Before sending data to the sink, data processing and data aggregation may be performed at the coordinator. Tier 3 represents Extra-WBANs in which the sink(s) send the collected data to the healthcare giver organizations using internet or any other network infrastructure.

A comprehensive survey on WBAN requirements and network technologies may be found in [17],[4],[16].

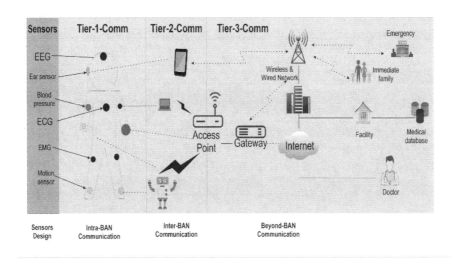

FIGURE 4.2: Three-tier WBAN architecture

4.2.1   BAN Design Aspects

Medical monitoring applications have specific hardware and network requirements [25], which are listed in the following.

1. WBANs allow the sensors to be deployed in, on or around a human body; so, 2 to 5 metre range is enough.

2. In a small deployment range, there may be a large number of sensors or actuators for health monitoring applications.

3. The WBAN standardisation group expects not more than 256 devices per network.

4. There will be interference due to transmissions by different sensors. There will be interferences due to transmissions by WBAN sensors and transmissions by other sources. Such interferences should be minimised to ensure reliable wireless communication.

5. Transmission of heath data must be timely and reliable.

6. Error detection and Error correction methods must be intrinsic to WBAN standards.

7. Different applications have different QoS requirements. So, QoS must be adaptible.

8. Latency must be lower than 125 milli second for medical applications.

9. Jitter reduces reliable transmision; so, it has to be within limits.

10. WBAN has to support different types of traffic: periodic and burst traffic.

11. Emergency traffic must take priority over normal messages on the network.That is, traffic may be continuous, periodic, or non-periodic and bursty.

12. Different applications need different data rates. In [5], bit rates and QoS requirements of different applications are mentioned. For example, applications for deep brain simulation needs a bit rate of 320 kbps or less while ECG, EEG and EMG applications require bit rates of 192 kbps, 86.4 kbps and 1.536 Mbps respectively. Glucose level monitors need data rates of 1kbps or less but capsule endoscopes and audio streaming need a data rate of 1 Mbps. Most of these applications require a delay of less than 250 micro second and a Bit Error Rate of 10^{-10} or less.

13. In-body environment plays a crucial role. Path loss in the transmission medium is always an important parameter in wireless communications. Obstacles between the transmitter and receiver increase this loss even further. The problem in WBAN is more serious, as the signal has to propagate through human tissues.

14. The body is a medium for communication of radio waves. Losses during propagation happen as power is absorbed into the tissue, and as a result, heat is generated. Human tissue mostly consists of water; so, significant attenuation of radio waves takes place when they propagate through a human body. Specific absorption rate (SAR) is used to determine the amount of power lost due to heat dissipation as a result of absorption in the tissue. Compared to propagation through a vacuum, an additional 3035 dB loss is noticed in transmission through human tissue. Moreover, human tissue is senitive to heat. So, WBAN communication should consider this aspect as well.

15. WBAN must be able to be interoperable with devices working on different types of networks.

16. Protection of privacy of the transmitted data and integrity of received information have to be ensured.

4.2.2   WBAN Sensors

Sensors in BANs are used in or around the body to collect signals of physical activities or of physiological conditions. Sensors send data as analog or digital signals, and then they are transmitted to the micro computing unit (MCU) for further processing. Some form of specialised pre-processing or filtering can also be implemented as algorithms in the MCU.

Microelectromechanical systems (MEMS) technology has played a significant role in implementing wearable sensor devices aimed at physiological and biokinetic user monitoring. These sensors may not necessarily be related to medical diagnosis and treatment. They reduce the importance of users' dependence on direct monitoring at hospitals, and thus lead to reduction of medical services and health-care costs.

Some sensor devices are implanted in the human body. Such implanted sensors jeopardise the health of users, and therefore, this practice is less preferred. Health hazards related to implanted sensors are manifold. These sensors may be rejected by the body; the sensor may even malfunction because of chemical reactions with the body tissues. To reduce such hazards, size and the biocompatibility of such sensors with human tissue is the greatest concern. Antenna design of such sensors is also very crucial. These antennas have to consume extremely low power, propagate signals efficiently, and even recover from unexpected errors.

4.2.3   Technologies for WBAN

A WBAN is a short-range wireless network. Many protocols such as Bluetooth, ZigBee, WiFi, IEEE 802.15.6 can be used to deploy WBAN.

4.2.3.1   Bluetooth and Bluetooth LE

Bluetooth is basically an IEEE 802.15.1 standard. This is also called WPAN (wireless personal area network). Bluetooth technology [18] was designed to provide a secured network for short-range wireless communications with much less power consumption. Devices supporting Bluetooth operate in the 2.4 GHz industrial, scientific and medical band (ISM). In order to mitigate interference, they use frequency hopping among seventy-nine 1 MHz channels at a nominal rate of 1600 hops/sec. Bluetooth technology supports three classes of devices. Bluetooth coverage ranges from 1 m to 100 m. It supports various transmission powers ranging from 1 mW to 100 mW with a 3 Mbps data rate. Bluetooth devices can communicate with each other under non-light-of-sight (NLOS) conditions. Applications between WBAN servers or applications between a WBAN and a personal computer are most appropriate for using Bluetooth protocol. The Bluetooth LE system is a lower current consumption version. Its maximum transmission range is 30 metre. The Bluetooth LE is suitable for applications with lower bit rates. The target applications include sports equipment and monitoring devices, speedometers, heart rate meters, pedometers, weight scales, glucose meters, blood pressure monitors, pulse oximeters, remote controls, tyre pressure monitoring, keyless entry, watch/wrist wearable devices.

Bluetooth LE operates in the 2.45 GHz ISM band, in which forty channels are defined. Width of each channel is 2 MHz. Since Bluetooth is a popular technology, it is a good choice for many WBAN applications. Recent tablets and mobile phones support dual-mode Bluetooth. Some monitoring devices, such as heart rate belts, support Bluetooth LE. Some of these are also available on the market. Bluetooth LE cannot support multihop communication and does not scale well. These are the primary shortcomings of Bluetooth LE.

4.2.3.2 ZigBee and WLAN

ZigBee is an IEEE 802.15.4 standard for wireless telecommunications [19]. It is designed for controls and sensors. ZigBee network is well known for its low power consumption. If the standby mode is effectively utlised, ZigBee-enabled devices can have a life span of several years. So, applications that require low energy consumption, low data rate, and secure networking are the main users of Zigbee networks. This makes this protocol useful for harsh or isolated conditions. The following three frequency bands are utilised by devices that support ZigBee: 868 MHz, 915 MHz, and 2.4 GHz. Therefore, ZigBee devices (particularly using 2.4 GHz) interfere with devices connected in wireless local area network (WLAN). This is why ZigBee cannot be chosen for WBAN. Moreover, ZigBee is not suitable for many real time WBAN applications, as the data rate of ZigBee-based devices is rather low.

WiFi is an IEEE 802.11 a/b/g/n/ac standard for wireless local area networks (WLAN). WiFi runs in ISM bands 2.4 GHz and 5 GHz. It has a coverage of 100 meter. If users are connected in ad hoc mode, or to an access point (AP), they are able to transfer data at broadband speed. If devices need very high-speed wireless connectivity and need to transfer data at a very high rate, WiFi is particularly suitable for them. Video conferencing, voice calls, and video streaming are typical WLAN applications. All smart phones, laptops, and tablets are integrated with WiFi connectivity. But WiFi consumes a lot of power. High energy-consumption is the most significant disadvantage of this technology. Thus, it cannot be adopted for WBAN.

4.2.3.3 WBAN standard

IEEE 802.15.6 is known as the WBAN standard. It supports communications inside and around a human body. Non-medical and medical applications, such as sports, environment monitoring, and eHealthcare monitoring use this protocol for communication.

The features of the physical layer of WBANs are different from those of wireless sensor networks or wireless ad-hoc networks. It is seen that nodes on the back of the patient and on the patient's chest cannot communicate with each other. Similarly, when a person sits on a chair, no communication may be possible between the chest and the ankle. The strength of the received signals is greatly influenced by the relative movement of the body parts. If the arms are moved in such a way that they obstruct the line between the two antennas, received signal is considerably attenuated. IEEE 802.15.6 standard supports three physical-layer standards to cater to all these needs.

Each physical-layer standard uses different frequency bands for data transmission. The maximum data rate supported is 10 Mbps. The first physical layer standard is narrowband (NB) which operates in the range of 400 MHz, 800 MHz, 900 MHz, 2.3 GHz, and 2.4 GHz bands. Another standard is human body communication (HBC). This operates at 50 MHz range. The third standard, known as ultra wideband (UWB) technology, operates between 3.1 GHz - 10.6 GHz. This standard supports high bandwidth in short range communication.

The transmission range cannot exceed 3 metres for applications within the body. For inter-body applications, transmission range is at least 3 metre. The topology of the network may be a star or a tree of at most a 2-hops.

MAC layer.

Although different physical-layer protocols are proposed for WBAN, only one single MAC protocol is proposed. As mentioned earlier, WBAN has to support various applications having different data flow types and data rates. Each application is characterised by its own performance requirements. So, the MAC protocol is flexible and supports both contention-based and contention-free access techniques.

One of the following three access modes can be selected by a BAN coordinator: beacon mode with superframes, also known as beacon periods, non-beacon mode with superframes, or non-beacon mode without superframes. In the first mode, the coordinator sends beacon packets to establish a common time base. Beacon packets specify the start of an active beacon period. This divides each active superframe (SF) into different access phases such as exclusive access phase (EAP), random access phase (RAP), managed access period (MAP), and Contention Access Period (CAP). These phases are ordered and the their specific durations are also defined. EAP is used only for transmitting emergency data. During EAP, RAP, and CAP, nodes use the CSMA/CA or Slotted ALOHA methods. In the MAP, actvities such as, scheduling intervals, or polling nodes are undertaken by the coordinator.

In the non-beacon mode with superframes, a coordinator has only a MAP in any SF. The coordiator organises access to the medium for the MAP phase in the first mode. In the last mode, a node may consider any time interval as a part of EAP1 or RAP1. A node contends for allocation using CSMA/CA-based random access.

Thus, the standard proposes several techniques for channel access, which makes it very flexible. But selection of the best option to produce optimal throughput, latency etc. for an application remains a challenging task.

The standard also supports three levels of security. Level 0 is meant for communications that can be unsecured. It provides no mechanism to ensure message authenticity, integrity, confidentiality and privacy. At level 1, messages are transmitted in secured authenticated but not encrypted frames. So, authentication and integrity validation are supported, but confidentiality is not supported in this level. At level 2, authentication as well as encryption are considered. As a result, this is the most secure transmission condition in which a part of message security, replay protection are provided.

4.2.4   Network Layer

We have already mentioned that features of WBAN are different from those of other wireless networks. Consequently design and development of efficient routing protocols for WBANs is a challenging task. A lot of research has been done for developing energy-efficient routing algorithms for ad hoc networks and WSNs. But those solutions do not meet the specific requirements of WBANs, as the characteristics of WSN and WBAN are different. An extensive survey of WBAN routing protocols may be found in [2]

The existing WBAN routing algorithms may be categorised as temperature-aware routing protocols, cluster-based routing protocols, QoS-aware routing protocols, cross-layered routing protocols etc. QoS aware routing protocols employ different components for measuring individual QoS parameters. Hence, they are modular-based protocols. QoS-aware FW, RL-QRP, LOCAL-MOR, QPRD, QPRR, Multihop, ENSA are some examples of QoS-aware routing protocols. Some well-known temperature aware routing protocols are: TARA, LTR, ALTR, LTRT, HPT, RAIN, TSHR, M-ATTEMPT, TMQoS, RE-ATTEMPT. HIT and ANYBODY are examples of cluster-based routing protocols. Some well-known cross layer routing algorithms are: WASP, CICADA, TICOSS, Biocomm, and Biocomm-D.

In this section, we shall discuss two routing protocols: one from the class of QoS-aware and the other from the thermal-aware class.

QoS-Aware peering routing for delay-sensitive data (QPRD) protocol [15] classifies the patient's data packets into two classes: ordinary packets (OP) and delay sensitive Packets (DSP). There are seven modules or components in the QPRD architecture. The MAC receiver component receives data from different nodes. The packet classifier component classifies packets as data or Hello packets, and chooses the best path for the packet.. The task of the delay module is to observe different types of delays and to forward the results to the network layer. The network layer computes the node delay. The hello protocol component is responsible for sending/receiving the hello packets. The routing service components receives the data packets from the layers above the network layer. The task of the QoS-aware queuing module is to forward the received data packets to their corresponding queue. Hello packets and the data packets are stored in a queue on a first-come-first-served (FCFS) basis by the MAC transmitter module. It transmits these packets using the CSMA/CA.

Increase in temperature of the body tissues around the implanted sensor nodes is a serious health hazard. So, controlling this rise of temperature is the major intention of all temperature-aware WBAN routing protocols. M-ATTEMPT [12] is an energy-efficient and thermal-aware routing protocol for WBANs that reduces temperature rise in the nodes, and at the same time, reduces the delay of the critical and sensitive data.

In this protocol, the sink node (base station) is assumed to be placed at the center while nodes with high data rates are deployed at less mobile body parts. To transmit data packets that are critical or query-driven, the sensor nodes transmit data packets directly to the sink node by increasing their transmission power. However, non-critical data packets are transmitted using multi-hop communication. All critical or query-driven data packets are sent to the sink first. Only then, ordinary data packets can be transmitted.

If two or more routes are available, the route with a lower hop-count is chosen. If two or more next-hop neighbor nodes have the same hop-count, the neighbour node which needs less energy to transfer the packet to the sink is chosen. M-ATTEMPT defines a threshold beyond which the temperature of a node is not allowed to rise. If the temperature at any node is more than the threshold, the node is called a hotspot, and the hotspot breaks all links with its neighbour nodes. It may so happen that the temperature at a node reaches the threshold after receiving a data packet. Then this node sends that packet back to the previous node. The previous node marks node from which the packet has returned as a hotspot.

There are four phases in the scheme proposed by M-ATTEMPT. They are: initialisation, routing, scheduling, and data transmission. In the initialization phase, all the nodes broadcast the hello packet. In the routing phase, those routes are selected which have lower hop-counts. In the scheduling phase, time division multiple access (TDMA) schedule is created by the sink node for all sensor nodes. The sensor nodes send data to the sink node during the data transmission phase.

4.2.5   Inter-WBAN Interference

According to the WBAN IEEE 802.15.6 standard, a system may consist of 10 coexisting WBANs and in each WBAN, there may be a maximum of 256 sensors. The standard demands that such a system must function efficiently within a transmission range of 3 metres. As per the standard, nodes in a single WBAN may use several access methods and can avoid interference. So, intra-WBAN communication may not have the problem of interference. However, a WBAN will interfere with other WBANs if they are in their mutual coverage area. Signals from a device on a person external to the WBAN may interfere with the signal between two devices on one person. These two signal-generating bodies are not synchronised. And the network topology is dynamic because of body movement. So, these links are not correlated and statistically independent. Thus, inter-WBAN interference becomes an important issue to be handled.

Fig. 4.3 shows the different types of interference in WBANs.

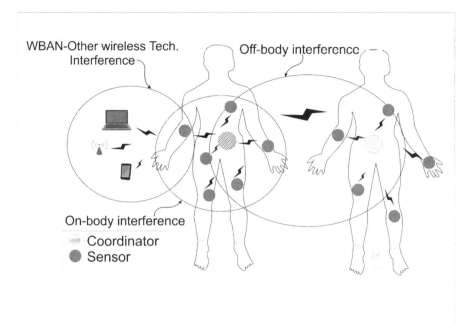

FIGURE 4.3: Inter-WBAN interference

There are two basic approaches for inter-WBAN intereference mitigation. One is by controlling the power and the other is by selecting proper channels. Many researchers used the power control method which are based on reinforcement learning or which uses game theoretic and fuzzy logic approaches [13]. These approaches try to maximise the achievable throughput and mitigate inter-network interference with minimum power consumption. Learning methods dynamically discover the environment and learn the best model to minimise energy consumption. In certain cases, learning-based algorithms perform better than the game theoretic or neuro-fuzzy approaches, but the computational overhead or convergence of learning methods remain unpredictable.

It has been seen that body posture has a significant contribution to path loss. [6] prposes an approach that reduces interferance due to body posture to achieve optimal power assignment. The authors use a range for RSSI values to obtain the right balance between energy consumption and packet loss. This scheme [6] tries to predict the posture position using the two most recently transmitted power RSSI data samples. The authors have not considered more samples, as that will take more time than the duration in which a person stays in a specific posture.

4.3   Crowdsourcing

Crowdsourcing may be termed as the activity in which organisations, in general, obtain services in the form of ideas, sources of data or information, or solutions to problems, among other things. The services would be obtained from a large, relatively open and often rapidly evolving group of Internet users [23]. The term *crowdsourcing* was coined in 2005 by Jeff Howe and Mark Robinson, to describe how businesses were using the Internet to "outsource work to the crowd". It was also mentioned in Howe's blog that the "crucial prerequisite is the use of the open call format and the large network of potential labourers."

Crowdsourcing can also be considered a type of participatory activity that happens online. For the activity to happen, a flexible open call for a task and voluntary efforts in answering the call are essential. The task may be simple or complex. Regardless of its complexity, the *crowd* is expected to share knowledge, experience, or work, whichever is applicable. They participate voluntarily, maybe for self-satisfaction, for social or economic recognition or development of individual skills, and so on.

Crowdsourcing is now gaining popularity. One of the causes is said to be the realisation of the companies that consumers are now all-powerful. Hence it seems to be a good move to involve them as partners and get their insights to the companies' advantage [14]. A few well known examples [14] are cited below.

In 2014, McDonalds came up with an idea to ask their customers to submit ideas for the types of burgers they would like to find in the store. The users would create their burgers online and the rest of the country could vote for the best ones.

Lego, the world-renowned toy company, also indulged themselves in crowdsourcing by allowing users to design new products, and at the same time, tested the demand for these products. Any user could submit a design and other users would vote. The idea with the most votes would eventually be produced and the creator would be rewarded.

Airbnb is one of the most well-known examples of successful crowdsourcing. Airbnb is a travel website that allows individuals to let out their homes to travelers across the world. Airbnbs business model is based on crowdsourcing. They also worked in joint collaboration on a crowdsourcing project that required filmmakers to create video content on homes or places to stay. The winners were also rewarded.

As is evident, there are different ways of incorporating crowdsourcing into business models. If someone wants to start a new company, or is looking for some marketing for his/her company or a company that wants to engage more with customers, then crowdsourcing may be one of the viable options.

We also find several crowdsourcing platforms [3] that help an idea take shape. Idea Bounty, OpenIdeo, and Innocentive are few platforms that allow creating discussions, getting help on project ideas, connecting with solution seekers, and so on. There are platforms that are meant for graphic and product design. Cad Crowd focuses on CAD modules. 99Designs, an artistic platform, is focused on graphic design. CrowdSpring allows freelancers to submit their solutions after someone posts his/her requirements. DesignCrowd lets one find designers using filters.

Still other platforms that are out there offer a broader range of crowd-sourced services. Microworkers is there for micro tasks such as signing up for a website, or completing a survey. mTurk, run by Amazon also does microtasks, like answering surveys, or commenting on blogs, among other such tasks. crowdSPRING is an online marketplace. It provides creative services which are crowdsourced from a large number of graphic designers and writers based in different countries. oDesk.com helps one find profiles for web developers, software and development designers, and such. In Elance, one can post a job and request and wait for interviews.

India has her own crowdsourcing platforms [9], namely Bitgiving, Crowdera, DreamWallets, FuelADream, FundDreamsIndia, Milaap, and Rang De. These platforms are involved in activities like fundraising for social causes, entrepreneurial efforts, sports, social enterprises, startups, and non-profit organisations. Some of these platforms also provide micro-cost loans to rural people or rural entrepreneurs across the country, or funding for creative projects like stand-up comedy, or film production.

Now we will focus on crowdsourcing for healthcare applications [11]. Office of the National Coordinator (ONC) for Health Information Technology of U.S. Department of Health and Human Services, supports crowdsourcing in healthcare. One of their initiatives is Crowds Care for Cancer, which is aimed towards development of innovative information management tools and applications. This includes managing the transition to primary care for speciality care survivors. Most important resources for these tools are healthcare providers and a patient support network. Generally, the platforms are compliant with the Health Insurance Portability and Accountability Act.

Crowdsourcing is also used for social and behavioural research in public health. Crowdsourced data samples will differ demographically, hence they have to be used for very specific purposes. Crowdsourced health-research studies are a pointer towards participatory health, where people use health social networks, crowdsourcing applications, smartphone health applications, and personal health records.

Some of the early discussions of medicine 2.0 or health 2.0 [21] focused on the deployment of social media (e.g., blogs, podcasts, tagging, search, wikis, video) by healthcare actors to improve collaboration and to personalise healthcare. The concept of *participatory medicine* is a direction towards healthcare personalisation. This was introduced in 2010. The aim was to focus on active participation by individuals. This may pave the way for personalised healthcare by utilising individual experiences, and needs. Crowdsourcing in health is generally reflected in researcher-organised and patient-organised crowdsource studies.

PatientsLikeMe (PLM) [10], is one of the operators of crowdsourced health research studies. PLM can boast of having one of the largest open patient registries and online health social networks (more than 125,000 members in 1000 condition-based communities as of January 2012). Members may enter demographic information. There will be other patients that may match a particular member's demographic and clinical characteristics. Thus a member will be able to find these patients like himself or herself. Members are also allowed to track their treatments, symptoms, and outcomes. Some crowdsourcing applications are based on questionnaires also. It seems that the personal connection that an individual has to health has made crowdsourced health research distinct from other similar research activities. In fact, apart from providing data about himself (crowdsourced data), a patient also becomes a part of the data analysis, leading to inferences that in turn prove to be helpful for the community.

Much of the available information in crowdsourced health research studies and health crowdsourcing sites is self-reported. Hence, whether the participant actually has the reported condition or the information provided is real, cannot be verified. Another point to ponder is whether the patients themselves are able to reliably report their own conditions or point towards a possible diagnosis. Another issue is that crowdsourced study members are like-minded participants, and so, they may not always represent the target population. This can result in either too homogeneous or too heterogeneous populations, and groups with high intra-individual variance, as well as small sample sizes. So, the results may not be statistically significant.

With the advent of different technologies, participatory health initiatives (self-tracking devices, smartphone applications, online personal health records, social networks on health, and health-research studies based on crowdsourcing) are on the rise. Individuals are keen to join studies conducted by researchers or research groups. People are also taking initiatives in designing such studies and conducting these.

Crowdsourcing is low in cost but high in speed. The data size grows at scales of magnitude much higher than before. It has the potential of discovering novel patterns in such large data sets, apart from the possibility of testing (almost real-time in nature) and applications of new medical findings.

4.4 Social Network

A *social network* may be considered to be a website that aims towards bringing people together, in a virtual sense. People are able to share ideas and interests, get to know each other, and make new friends. This type of non-physical collaboration and sharing is termed social media. Social networking applications uses the association between individuals and facilitate them further for creating new connections.

A 2016 statistics find the following few popular social media sites:

- Facebook: This is the biggest social media network. The number of users is quite large.

- Twitter: This social medial platform has millions of users whose posts started with the limit of 140 characters, that have now doubled.

- LinkedIn: This is the most popular social media site for professional networking.

- Google+: It has also become one of the largest social media sites in no time.

- YouTube: Among the video-based social media websites, this is the largest and most popular.

- Tumblr: Tumblr is the platform for visual social media.

- Flickr: Flicker is an online image and video-hosting platform.

- WhatsApp: WhatsApp Messenger is a cross-platform instant messaging client for small devices including smartphones, PCs, and tablets.

- Quora: Quora is there to satisfy human inquisitiveness.

Social network sites and social media are typical online social platforms. As seen from the different sites mentioned above, the aims of social media sites are collaboration among individuals and the exchange of information, to name a few. People with specific objectives may also take part in any such media. Organisations therefore can also participate in social media sites with an aim towards increasing their client base. Nowadays, almost all small businesses, including various shops and publishing houses target social media, and quite expectedly, they are getting more clients.

The health industry has found a new friend in social networks. It is using these sites to support, promote, and increase the spread of information and data, ranging from clinical healthcare to public health campaigns. This is done in order to improve both personal and community health practices. Social media has provided the opportunity to share preventative information. They have provided the opportunity to create support structures. The support structures, in turn, not only helps to track personal health but also builds up further support networks. These newly formed patient-to-patient networks provide the much needed extended support post-diagnosis.

The social media sites allow participants to share interests and opinions as well as social interactions. The use of these platforms is increasing in leaps and bounds. Social networking sites may play a role for health-related issues in some of the following ways: (1) The presence of health organisations on these sites makes them more approachable and accessible; (2) Patients with chronic or typical diseases may connect with each other via these sites and (3) Caregivers for critical patients may also form groups to share and exchange crucial information.

Until now, the health research literature has focused on social network sites either as tools to deliver health care, or to analyse Web health content. However, evidence shows that health research is now using social networks in many forms [7].

It is now seen that medical practitioners have started developing an interest in online interacting with patients. Some physicians are using social media, including LinkedIn, blogs, Twitter, and Facebook. They find the media helpful in providing and enhancing the communication with patients.

Studies show that medical practitioners use social media for both personal as well as professional reasons. Thus, social media sites for healthcare professionals have also cropped up. Physician-only site like Sermo allows doctors to discuss treatment options and ask for expert advice. A large number of U.S. healthcare professions have found Doximity to be useful as it sets up an indirect way for patients to contact them [22]. The concept is to use a national database where accounts of U.S. physicians are created with demographic and contact information.

Healthcare professionals may not always use social media for direct patient care. However, social media usage is slowly being accepted by healthcare professionals and facilities. For example, Georgia Health Sciences University has provided patients with access to 'WebView', which allows patients to communicate with their doctors for queries on symptoms or diagnosis or prescription refills [22].

Microblogs, as the terminology suggests, is shorter form of blogs. Hence, microblog is meant to provide a concise form of exchange of information, carried out via social media. This allows users to post numbers of short messages or updates over a short period. Twitter is one of the most important and popular among the microblogging platforms. There are more than 140 reported uses for Twitter in health care. Some of them are: food safety alert, pain management, issuing asthma alert, opinion sharing by physicians, tracking disease-specific trends, and so on.

Now we would like to focus on how data regarding health information in social media can be utilised. In 2009, the U.S. Centers for Disease Control and Prevention took advantage of social media posts made by users regarding the H1N1 virus. It used posts that mention possible symptoms and also claims of possible outbreak of the H1N1 virus. This was done to raise awareness among the public. The general public accessed information on how to identify symptoms of the virus and thereby avoid certain locations prone to possible outbreak. The government was quick to mobilise resources and prevent mass panic. The CDC also created the Predict the Influenza Season Challenge competition. Participants tried to develop modeling tools that could predict seasonal flu activity based on information gathered from social media networks [1].

As mentioned above in this subsection, social media networks allow interaction of patients with each other. As an example, patients diagnosed with depression share their thoughts and are ready to connect with other similar patients and doctors. Researchers are of the opinion that monitoring these networks in real-time will provide more accurate data and information than traditional annual surveys. The methods used to collect information may include identifying (and cross-referencing) depression-related and associated key words in a post [1]. Analysis of this huge data would contribute to society by screening people who may have different attitudes towards life, so that they may be properly counseled.

Generally, consumers voice their concerns regarding different health issues on social media sites. One of these concerns is adverse drug reactions. Agencies may monitor social networking sites for such comments with an aim to enhance the alert system regarding the effects of the drug.

In [8] the authors discuss an approach to integrating health data sources available on social sites, and presenting them so as to be easily understandable by physicians, healthcare staff, and patients. At the implementation level, data is stored as RDF (resource description framework) triples, which provides: (1) flexibly describing data with heterogeneous features; (2) homogeneous data access; (3) the opportunity for data linkage and semantic enrichment. The integration model is then used as the basis for developing a set of analytics which is part of a system called Social InfoButtons. The prototype system provides patients, public health officials, and healthcare specialists with a unified view of health-related information. It provides the capability of exploring the current data along multiple dimensions, such as time and geographical location.

One of the main concerns, however, is how much you can depend on all this information found on different social media sites. Quality and reliability issues are the concerns of the day. Authors of medical information on social media sites are often unknown or rarely identifiable. Also, it may not be possible to track or refer the medical information, and it may be an incomplete information lacking the formality of terminologies. Apart from this, patient data privacy is always an issue to deal with.

HIPAA, as modified by the Health Information Technology for Economic and Clinical Health (HITECH) act, governs the permitted use and disclosure of patient information by covered entities, like healthcare professionals and hospitals. The HITECH act lays down in detail the privacy-breach notification requirements [22].

The data size, although vast, can result in either underestimating or overestimating the correctness of a situation. In such situation, policy level errors may happen and the public may be inadvertently affected. For example misleading information regarding the spread of a disease may go out to the public. Therefore, during health crises the health agencies and other organisations have to responsibly manage misinformation. Proper steps regarding issuing of advisories and circulars have to adopted on urgent basis.

However, medical practitioners, researchers, and other stakeholders must consider the potential benefits of using social media. This is because of the fact that,the media is able to provide timely data that may be utilised to obtain the trends and patterns in health. To determine and predict health trends, syndromic surveillance can readily use information shared over social media sites.

With the implementation of social media as part of a broader IT strategy, public health leaders, working with their international counterparts and the private sector, can proactively develop solutions leading to further advances in research and development. Continuous advancement in mobile health (mHealth) that will unveil new questions about data sharing and privacy has been predicted. This will be crucial and interesting as we enter the era of personalised medicine.

4.5   Chapter Notes

Acquisition of data is one of the major tasks in any application. And for healthcare applications, the data becomes the Big Heath Data. Since there are different types of healthcare applications, it is only natural that acquisition techniques have to be different. This chapter discusses WBAN, and the role of Crowdsourcing and Social Networks in data acquisition. Besides healthcare applications, depending on the types of applications there may be other data acquisition techniques that are not within the scope of this book.

References

[1] Altug Akay, Andrei Dragomir, and Bjorn-Erik Erlandsson. Mining social media big data for health. *IEEE Pulse*, 16(7), 2015.

[2] Javed Iqbal Bangash, Abdul Hanan Abdullah, Mohammad Hossein Anisi, and Abdul Waheed Khan. A Survey of Routing Protocols in Wireless Body Sensor Networks. *Sensors*, pages 1322–1357, 2014.

[3] Hannah Bensoussan. Top 13 crowdsourcing platforms to design your product. https://www.sculpteo.com/blog/2016/10/19/13-best-crowdsourcing-platforms-for-product-design/, 2016.

[4] Min Chen, Sergio Gonzalez, Athanasios Vasilakos, Huasong Cao, and Victor C. M. Leung. Body area networks: A survey. *Mobile Networks and Applications*, 16(2):171–193, 2011.

[5] C. Cordeiro. Use cases, applications, and requirements for bans. *IEEE802.15-07-0564-00-0 BAN*, 2007.

[6] J. Dong and D. Smith. Reinforcement learning in power control games for internetwork interference mitigation in wireless body area networks. In *Proceedings of the IEEE International Conference on Communication, ICC*, pages 5676–5681. IEEE, 2014.

[7] Fahdah Alshaikh et al. Social network sites as a mode to collect health data: A Systematic Review. *J Med Internet Res*, 16(7), 2014.

[8] Xiang Ji et al. Linking and using social media data for enhancing public health analytics. *Journal of Information Science*, 16(7), 2016.

[9] Pratibha Goenka. A list of 15 crowdfunding platforms in India. https://in.thehackerstreet.com/15-crowdfunding-platforms-india/, 2017.

[10] Sunil Gupta and Jason Riis. Patientslikeme: An Online Community of Patients. https://www.hbs.edu/faculty/Pages/item.aspx?num=40054, 2012.

[11] Chris Hoffmann. The 8 categories of crowdfunding in healthcare. https://medcitynews.com/2015/01/8-categories-crowdsourcing-healthcare/, 2015.

[12] N. Javaid, Z. Abbas, M. S. Fareed, Z. A. Khan, and N. Alrajeh. M-attempt: A new energy-efficient routing protocol for wireless body area sensor networks. *Procedia Comput*, 19:224–231, 2013.

[13] R. Kazemi, R. Vesilo, E. Dutkiewicz, and R. P. Liu. Reinforcement learning in power control games for internetwork interference mitigation in wireless body area networks. In *Proceedings of the International Symposium on Communicaton and Information Technology*, ISCIT, pages 256–262. IEEE, 2012.

[14] Kathryn Kearns. 9 great examples of crowdsourcing in the age of empowered consumers. http://tweakyourbiz.com/marketing/2015/07/10/9-great-examples-crowdsourcing-age-empowered-consumers/, 2015.

[15] Z. A. Khan, S. Sivakumar, W. Phillips, and B. A. Robertson. Qos-aware routing protocol for reliability sensitive data in hospital body area networks. *Procedia Comput*, 19:171–179, 2013.

[16] B. Malik and V. R. Singh. A survey of research in WBAN for biomedical and scientific applications. *Health and Technology*, 3(3):227–235, 2013.

[17] Samaneh Movassaghi, Mehran Abolhasan, and Justin Lipman. Wireless body area networks: A survey. *IEEE Communications Surveys and Tutorials*, 16(3):1658–1686, 2014.

[18] Specification of the Bluetooth System version 4.0. Bluetooth sig, 2010.

[19] IEEE 802.15.4 Standard. Part 15.4: Wireless Medium Access Control (mac) and Physical Layer (phy) Specifications for Low-rate Wireless Personal Area Networks (LR-WPANs), 2006.

[20] IEEE 802.15.6 Standard. IEEE standard for local and metropolitan area networks part 15.6: Wireless body area networks, 2012.

[21] Melanie Swan. Crowdsourced Health Research Studies: An Important Emerging Complement to Clinical Trials in the Public Health Research Ecosystem Monitoring. *J Med Internet Res*, 14(2), 2012.

[22] C. Lee Ventola. Social media and health care professionals: Benefits, risks, and best practices. *Pharmacy and Therapeutics*, 39(7), 2014.

[23] Wikpedia. Crowdsourcing. https://en.wikipedia.org/wiki/Crowdsourcing, 2017.

[24] Yang and Guang-Zhong (Ed.). *Body Sensor Networks*. Springer, 2014.

[25] B. Zhen, M. Patel, S. Lee, E. Won, and A. Astrin. Tg6 technical requirements document (trd). *IEEE p802. 15-08-0644-09-0006*, 2008.

5

Health Data Analytics

CONTENTS

5.1	Introduction	88
5.2	Artificial Neural Networks	90
	5.2.1 Model of an ANN	90
	5.2.2 Modes of ANN	92
	5.2.3 Structure of ANNs	93
	5.2.4 Training a Feedforward Neural Network	93
	5.2.5 ANN in Medical Domain	96
	5.2.6 Weakness of ANNs	97
5.3	Classification and Clustering	98
	5.3.1 Clustering via K-Means	99
	5.3.2 Some Additional Remarks about K-Means	100
5.4	Statistical Classifier: Bayesian and Naive Classification	102
	5.4.1 Experiments with Medical Data	104
	5.4.2 Decision Trees	106
	5.4.3 Clasical Indction of Decision Trees	108
5.5	Association Rule Mining (ARM)	111
	5.5.1 Simple Approach for Rule Discovery	112
	5.5.2 Processing of Medical Data	113
	5.5.3 Association Rule Mining in Health Data	113
	5.5.4 Issues with Association Rule Mining	114
5.6	Time Series Analysis	115
	5.6.1 Time Series Regression Models	116
	5.6.2 Linear AR Time Series Models	117
	5.6.3 Application of Time Series	120
5.7	Text Mining	120
	5.7.1 Term Frequency and Inverse Document Frequency	122
	5.7.2 Topic Modeling	123
5.8	Chapter Notes	124

5.1   Introduction

In the last few decades, an enormous amount of health data has been generated since the advent of new data sensing and acquisition technologies. Transformation of this data into knowledge by using appropriate analytical techniques is the next big challenge. Analysis of health data will exhibit the patterns hidden in the data. It may also help in creating personalised profiles that in turn may lead to discovering that the likelihood of a patient to suffer from a medical complication or disease in later years. Thus, effective analytical tools that can understand health data and discover and predict new facts have the potential to transform healthcare delivery systems from being reactive to become proactive. It is therefore natural that the use of analytics on healthcare data will grow in leaps and bounds in years to come.

Sources of healthcare data are various. For instance, the sensors, the images, the medical reports, the traditional electronic records, clinical notes, prescriptions are sources of health data. This data is collected in a variety of ways and represented in several forms and formats. This heterogeneity in the data collection and representation poses serious challenges in processing and analysing data. Each type of data has to be processed and analysed differently from the other type of data. Not only in processing and analysis, heterogeneity of data makes integration a formidable task. This integration, however, is an important task. Insights that can be obtained from the combined data may not be obtained by looking at a single source of the data. Recent advancements in data analysis methods have the potential to explore this huge amount of data in an integrated manner.

The field of healthcare is truly interdisciplinary in nature. Advances in electronics, information technology, biochemistry, and experience of medical practitioners - all these have enriched this field. Databases, data mining, information retrieval techniques help in healthcare delivery as much as the outcomes of medical researchers and healthcare practitioners. This interdisciplinary nature has its unique, peculiar challenges. Computer scientists and information technologists are not familiar with the concepts in the medical domain, whereas researchers and practitioners in the medical domain do not have necessary expertise in the field of data analytics. Without this symbiosis, much of medical data generated in so many ways cannot be processed using advanced analysis techniques.

Such a diversity often leads to independent research from completely distinct points of view. Those who work in the field of data analytics may invent methods and techniques for problems but they may not have access to real data from practical domains. Consequently, these novel methods and techniques have very limited practical use.

The sources for medical data are very heterogeneous. Different sources produce data with very different characteristics. As a result, various data analysis methods are to be applied to these heterogeneous data. Electronic health records (EHRs) are digital versions of patients' medical data. It contains comprehensive data related to a patient's care. This data includes demographics, symptoms, problems, medications, vital statistics, medical history, pathological test reports, X-Ray images, notes on progress, and billing information. Many EHRs are not limited to a patient's comprehensive medical history, They may contain additional information of a patient from a broader point of view.

Biomedical images obtained by magnetic resonance imaging (MRI), computed tomography (CT), positron emission tomography (PET), and ultrasound imaging are very useful data for patient monitoring and prognosis. But these images are varied, complex, and often noisy. Image processing is an established field in the disciplines of computer science and electronics. There are many standard algorithms for image segmentation, object detection, feature extraction, and classification. These general purpose, domain-independent techniques are now successfully customised for analysis of medical images to detect a number of diseases or understand their progression.

Sensor data, such as electrocardiograms (ECG) and electroencephalograms (EEG) have value for both real time and retrospective analysis. For critical healthcare such as patients in ICU or patients moving in ambulance, the data from sensors are used for real-time analysis. In such cases, any deviation from normal conditions results in generation of alerts or triggering of alarms. Sometimes sensor data are also useful for remote monitoring of patients. In remote monitoring applications, however, long-term analysis of various trends and patterns in the data may become more useful to predict some future problems. As sensors produce data continually, the amonut of data generated by them is enoromous. These applications necessitate the use of big data frameworks and corresponding analytic tools [3]. Since big data is relatively new, novel data analytical tools to process and analyse large volumes of data using the new paradigm of computing are only emerging. These methods and tools have the potential to revolutionise healthcare delivery systems that may help to reduce cost and improve efficiency.

To date, most of the patient's information is stored in clinical notes. These contain medical transcription which may be handwritten or entered by a data entry operator, or by the practitioner. These data form the backbone of much of healthcare data. They also form the richest source of information, But these notes are unstructured and stored in an unstructured format only, and therefore they are very difficult to analyse automatically. This is so because the notes written in a natural language have to be converted to a structured language that is extremely complex. Not only are these notes unstructured, they are heterogeneous, having diverse formats and contextual. Natural language processing (NLP) is a rich field of study in which several problems are addressed. These problems include shallow or full parsing, sentence segmentation, text categorisation, entity extraction, etc. But processing of medical information is significantly different from processing other texts.

Text mining methods and tools are also used in the medical domain. Text mining attempts to discover knowledge and pattern hidden in the data in the biomedical field. Such tools offer efficient ways to search, extract entities and events, combine, analyse and summarise textual data, thus supporting researchers in knowledge discovery and generation. There are many advantages of applying text mining methods and techniques in the medical domain. These techniques have the potential to discover useful knowledge in unstructured or semi-structured data. They can also discover even less-precisely defined entities and their associations. The cost of manually curating huge amount of text data available in the medical field is exorbitant. It may be possible to apply text mining methods to populate, update, and integrate this data in a useful manner. In addition, text mining has the promise to link textual evidences and generate hypotheses at a reduced cost.

So far, we have discussed the characteristics of health data generated from different sources. In this chapter, we shall discuss a few data analytics methods relevant for healthcare data. We shall discuss some data mining and machine learning models that have already been adapted to the healthcare domain. The methods that we shall discuss in this chapter include (i) some statistical methods such as linear regression, and Bayesian models, (ii) advanced methods in machine learning and data mining, such as decision trees and artificial neural networks, and (iii) text mining methods.

5.2 Artificial Neural Networks

An artificial neural network (ANN) [8] is a computational paradigm that is based on mathematical models resembling a human brain. The human brain comprises billions of neurons which are interconnected. Likewise, an ANN comprises many processing elements which are interconnected. Similar to a human brain, the processing elements can function in parallel. That is why ANNs are often referred to as connectionist systems, parallel distributed systems, or adaptive systems. ANNs are not controlled by a central node. Instead, all interconnected processing elements adapt to the flow of information according to certain rules. ANNs are applied to solve problems from various domains ranging from pattern recognition and classification to optimisation and data compression. Since the 1990s, ANNs have also been used in the field of health data, specifically for medical diagnosis [7].

5.2.1 Model of an ANN

A brief description of several ANN models and their applications in medical domain is available in [23]. As we have already mentioned, an ANN is composed of a large number of artificial neurons or processing elements. These artificial neurons are connected with weights. The network is also organised in layers. Each processing element (PE) has weighted inputs on which a transfer function is applied to produce an output. The overall function of an ANN is determined by the individual transfer functions of its neurons, and its architecture. In an ANN, the weights are parameters which can be adjusted. So, an ANN is called a parameterised system. An activation of an ANN is formed by the weighted sum of the inputs. Then, transfer functions are applied on these activation signals and an output is produced. Non-linearity of an ANN is brought about by the transfer functions.

The perceptron is a simple neuron model that accepts input signals coded as an input vector $X = (x_1, x_2, \cdots, x_n)$, where x_i is the signal from the i-th input. A synaptic weight is associated with each input signal coming from another neuron. Weights connected to the i-th neuron are represented by a vector $W_i = (w_1, w_2, \cdots, w_n)$. Let SUM denote the weighted sum of inputs as defined in the following.

$$SUM = \sum_{i=1}^{n} x_i w_i$$

The output y of a neuron is defined as an activation function f of the weighted sum of $n + 1$ inputs. By convention, if there are n inputs to the perceptron, the input $n + 1$ will be fixed to -1 and its weight is assigned some θ where θ is the value of the excitation threshold.

$$y = f(\sum_{i=1}^{n} x_i w_i)$$

A model of an perceptron is shown in Figure 5.1.

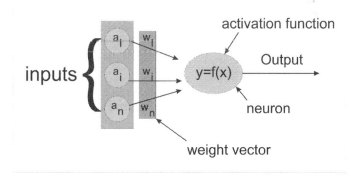

FIGURE 5.1: Model of an ANN

5.2.2   Modes of ANN

An artificial neural network works in two different modes: training and testing. During training, the ANN is provided with a set of known examples. As the training starts, the network tries to guess the output corresponding to the examples. Training is an iterative process during which the weights associated to the neurons change so that the outputs for all imputs become the most accurate. In other words, during the process of training, the network adapts itself until it achieves a stable configuration in which the outputs are satisfactorily correct. Learning in neural networks can be either supervised or unsupervised.

In supervised learning, the network is trained using a database that contains a number of examples where the input is provided along with their correct output. The objective is to tutor the network to associate the given input with the desired output. The network accepts each example in the training database as an input and produces an actual output. If the actual output differs from the desired output, the weights in the network are adjusted and the network is tried again. This continues till the output produced is adequately close to the expected output, or the network cannot improve its accuracy any more.

The final task of an ANN is to provide an output to an input it has not seen before, Thus, the performance of the machine may not be evaluated by observing how accurately the ANN can provide outputs of known inputs. The ANN should learn the underlying aspects of the input-output mapping and then generalises to new inputs.

In unsupervised learning, the ANN has to work without the supervision of a teacher. Even then, an ANN has two modes. During the training mode of an ANN under unsupervised learning, clusters are formed by combining input vectors of similar types. Each cluster represents a set of elements which have some common characteristics. When a new input pattern is provided to the ANN, it produces an output that shows the class corresponding to the new input pattern. In this case, there is no feedback from the environment to indicate whether the produced output is correct. Thus, in unsupervised learning, the ANN has to discover the features from the input data, and find out the pattern and the mapping from input to output.

In both supervised and unsupervised learning, after the network attains the expected accuracy, the training stage is said to be complete and the weights so obtained become fixed. The final state of the network is preserved and it is then used to produce outputs for inputs, previously not encountered. If the learning process of the ANN is satisfactory, it should be able to generalise. That is, the actual output produced by the network for unseen inputs should be almost as good as the outputs produced during the learning stage.

5.2.3 Structure of ANNs

Artificial neural networks are normally organised in terms of layers. Each layer in this network comprises an array of neurons or PEs. Neurons belonging to the same layer are not connected. Neurons belonging to consecutive layers are connected. Each neuron from layer i is connected to a neuron in layer $i + 1$. Multilayer perceptron (MLP) is a typical example of such a network (Figure 5.2). MLP networks may have many layers but they normally have three layers of PEs with only one hidden layer. The input layer is only responsible for receiving the external stimuli and for propagating it to the next layer. The task of the hidden layer is to process the input by using an activation function. The activation functions most commonly used are the step (Figure 5.3), sigmoid (Figure 5.4), and hyperbolic tangent (Figure 5.5) functions. The activation functions have to be differentiable.

The processing elements in the hidden layer produce outputs in turn that are fed to the neurons in the next layer. This adjacent layer could be the output layer itself or another hidden layer of processing elements. In this manner, information is propagated in the forward direction until an output is produced by the network.

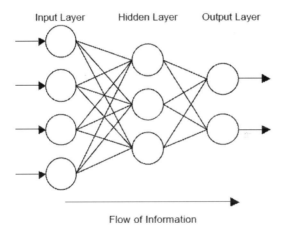

FIGURE 5.2: Structure of an ANN

5.2.4 Training a Feedforward Neural Network

Back propagation neural network (BPN) is a multilayer neural network comprising the input layer, at least one hidden layer, and the output layer. Error is calculated at the output layer by comparing the expected output and the actual output obtained. This error is propagated back towards the input layer.

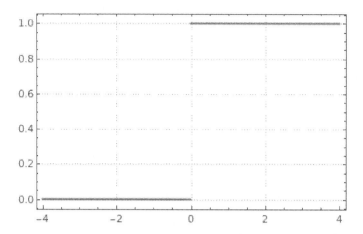

FIGURE 5.3: Step function

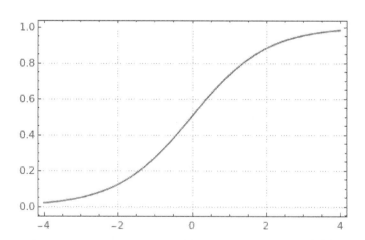

FIGURE 5.4: Sigmoid function

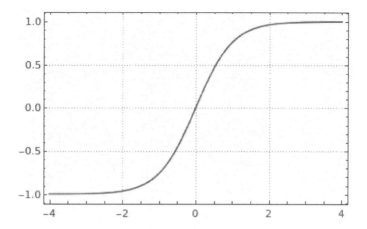

FIGURE 5.5: Hyperbolic tangent function

The architecture of BPN is shown in the Figure 5.6. The hidden layer and the output layer of a BPN have an additional input, called bias. The weight of bias is always 1. The BPN works in three phases. In the first phase, input signals are sent to the output layer. In the second phase, the error is back propagated from the output layer to the input layer. Weights are updated in the third phase.

The training algorithm can be formalized as shown in Algorithm 1. This algorithm is adapted from [26]

During training, the weights in a network are changed to minimise the difference between the output and input. The learning rule specifies the way in which these weights are modified. The most common rules are generalisations of the least mean square error (LMS) rule.

In supervised learning, a feedforward ANN is trained with examples of input-output pairs. For each input, an output is produced by the ANN. The error E is defined as the difference between the output o produced by the network and the expected output t.

$$E = \frac{1}{2} \sum_{1=1}^{n} (t - o)^2$$

Weights are adjusted so that the overall output error computed using the equation above can be minimised. This error E is propagated backwards from the output layer to the input. The weights in the ANN are changed or adjusted by a fraction d of E. Once the adjustments to the weights are made, examples are provided to the ANN once again. This process of computing error and adjusting weights are repeatedly carried out until the output becomes satisfactory or accuracy of the outputs in the ANN cannot be improved any further.

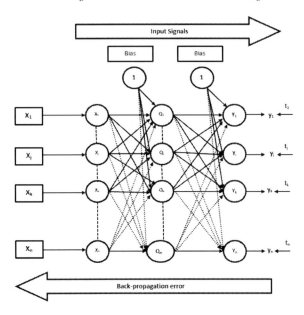

FIGURE 5.6: Architecture of a back propagation network

5.2.5   ANN in Medical Domain

A good survey on the use of ANN for medical image processing may be found in [24], [10]. Neural networks are established as good classifiers. They are also successfully used for function approximation. So, they have been successfully used in medical image processing. They are specifically used for preprocessing, segmentation, registration, and recognition. The process by which distinct datasets are transformed into one coordinate system is called image registration. Registration is required to compare, integrate, and fuse images from different measurements, which may be taken at different points in time using the same technique or obtained from different techniques such as MR, CT, ultrasound, and angiography. Medical image segmentation is a process used to divide an image into regions having uniform characteristics. Image segmentation is necessary in finding out the boundaries of organs and tumours. Thus, segmentation of medical images is very significant in identifying diseases, clinical research, and several such applications. Image segmentation and edge detection normally follow image registration and are two very important preprocessing steps in medical image processing.

The most popular ANN for medical image segmentation is a feedforward neural network. Fuzzy Gaussian basis neural networks, contextual neural networks, and probabilistic neural networks. Hybrid neural networks are also applied in segmentation of medical images.

For image reconstruction, Hopfield neural networks are the most popularly used ANN. Many other neural networks are also used to detect and recognise medical images.

Back propagation ANNs are used for mammography interpretation and diagnostic decision making [2], diagnosis of disease from ultrasound images of liver [12], differential diagnosis of interstitial lung disease [1], and many such applications.

One problem with ANNs is that the accuracy of prediction on data which was not used to train it may be low. The ability of ANNs to predict accurately when given data is not used during training is known as generalisation ability. If we combine many ANNs, the generalisation ability can be greatly enhanced. This approach of combining ANNs is known as an artificial neural network ensemble [25], [29]. An artificial neural network ensemble is composed of many ANNs that are trained for the same problem. The predictions of the individual ANNs are combined to produce the overall output. ANN ensembles have a better generalisation capability and increased stability than a single ANN. Ensemble ANNs have been successfully applied in medical diagnosis. It can be theoretically explained that ANN ensembles with a plurality consensus voting exhibit significantly more generalisation capability than a single ANN. In plural consensus voting, the classification obtained by the majority of the ANNs is accepted as the final result. It is proved that the average generalisation ability and the average ambiguity of the ANNs which make up an ensemble determines the generalisation ability of the ensemble as a whole.

Suppose that an ANN ensemble is used in cancer detection. Let the ensemble be built in two levels. The first-level ensemble is used to decide whether a cell is normal or cancerous. So, each individual ANN has two outputs indicating that a cell is either normal or a cancerous . The outputs of the individual ANNs in the ensemble have to be combined using some method. The second-level ensemble handles only cancerous cells. In the second level, each individual network has several outputs corresponding to various types of cancer. Plurality voting may be one way to combine the predictions of these individual ANNs. It is likely that the ANN ensemble has a low rate of false negative; i.e., ANN ensemble normally does not indicate a cancerous cells as a normal cell.

5.2.6   Weakness of ANNs

Artificial neural networks have been very successful in several fields, but they also suffer from several serious shortcomings.

There are many types of models for neural networks. Choosing the best neural network model and the corresponding architecture is a very difficult problem. In spite of some research work being carried out in the literature for model selection, no general guidelines exist for selecting a model given a task.

ANNs must be designed by trial and error. So, construction of an ANN model is a very time consuming process.

The addition of many hidden layers raises the problem of over-fitting the data; This means that the network learns too well in the training data session but generates worse results in the case of unknown inputs. Therefore, it is not necessary that minimising the error in the training dataset will always result in an ANN that generalises well.

Another problem with ANNs is that they are black-box in nature. Even if an artificial neural network works well, there is no analytical reasoning about how it works. We may find that for an input a corresponding output is produced. But how the output is reached cannot be explained and therefore its reliability is always questionable.

The next problem is that a human expert's knowledge and experience cannot be directly expressed in an ANN. Also, the construction of its topological structure is not easily amenable to formal analysis. Moreover, the weights of the ANN cannot be associated with any physical meaning. Because of these reasons, effective neural networks may be hard to design. Combining fuzzy technique with neural networks and processing fuzzy information by neural networks may overcome some of these shortcomings. In that case, neural networks becomes capable of expressing qualitative knowledge. The topological structure of the ANN and weights can be associated with physical meaning. Moreover, network initialisation becomes easier, local optimisation of network training can be avoided, and the stability of networks can be ensured.

In medical image processing, the amount of input data for training an ANN also poses a problem. In order to obtain high precision on data not used in training, the amount of data required during training is huge. Technology for the acquisition of medical images is advancing rapidly. Development of CAD schemes should also be at the same pace. Otherwise, obtaining a large amount of data for training for abnormal cases is very difficult. Without a large amount of data for normal and abnormal cases, the performance of ANNs will degrade.

5.3   Classification and Clustering

Clustering is logically dividing data into groups of objects having similar characteristics. Each such group is called a cluster. A cluster comprises objects that are similar among themselves and significantly different from objects belonging to other clusters. Clusters correspond to some hidden patterns that are inherent to data. Clustering [27] is an unsupervised machine learning technique, that has several significant applications in healthcare.

Suppose that a model is meant to forecast the probability that a patient will develop diabetes. In most cases, there will be a set of input attributes such as blood pressure, weight, age, etc. And there is a set of outputs which may be a label indicating whether a person has diabetes or not. It is possible to train a supervised classifier to learn the patterns of attributes associated with different possible outputs. Thereafter, when the trained classifier encounters a new patient, the classifier may be able to predict whether the new patient is diabetic or not. In this example, there is a training database that contains correct outputs for several inputs and thus, this is an example of supervised learning.

Assume that the input-output pairs of a training database are not available or that these pairs, even if present, are not reliable. In such a case, groups of people with diabetes and without diabetes have to be discovered only from the input values. In such cases, we must resort to unsupervised learning. Clustering helps us to discover a pattern in a collection of data if the training dataset is not present.

5.3.1   Clustering via K-Means

K-means is a classical method to solve clustering problems [13]. It is one of the simplest yet the most popular unsupervised learning algorithms. The goal of k-means clustering algorithm is to find the set of k clusters such that every data point is associated with the closest centre, and the sum of the distances of all such associations is minimised.

For example, suppose that we have the following points as shown in Figure 5.7. We like to group these points in three clusters. The k-means algorithm comprises four steps as described in the following:

Step 1: Initialise cluster centres.
Three points C_1, C_2 and C_3 are selected at random. These are identified to represent the cluster centres (shown in gray scale). See Figure 5.8.

Step 2: Cluster assignment.
The next step is to associate each point to a cluster depending on its distance from the already identified cluster centres. A point is assigned that cluster whose centre's distance from the point is the minimum. Consider the grey point A in Figure 5.9. We compute its distance d_1, d_2 and d_3 from C_1, C_2, and C_3, respectively. We find the minimum of these three distances, d_1, d_2, and d_3. In this case, the minimum distance is d_1. So, the point A is associated to the gray cluster and the point is coloured as gray.

The other points will be taken one by one and the same procedure is repeated. Thus, all points are assigned their clusters.

Step 3: Move cluster centres (centroids).
The next step is to update the cluster centers or centroids. In this example, the centre of the gray cluster is recomputed by calculating the centroid of all gray points. And the point C_1' becomes the new center for the gray cluster. In a similar manner, the new centers C_2' and C_3' may be computed for the hatched and exchequer clusters.

Step 4: Repeat the previous two steps until there is no change in clusters or

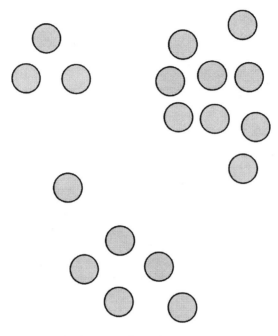

FIGURE 5.7: Set of points in 2D

the number of iterations are more than a fixed number. The final clusters for this example are shown in Figure 5.10.

How to choose the value of k is an important question. We can run the experiment using different values of k and find out the value of k for which good clusters are generated. If some clusters have a very small number of members, the value of k can be decreased. If the clusters are too large, the value of k may be increased. In order to find out the value of k algorithmically, we can cluster with increasing values of k and plot various metrics denoting the quality of the resulting clusters. Then, we can choose the value of k for best clustering.

5.3.2 Some Additional Remarks about K-Means

Since its invention, the k-means algorithm has been applied to many problems in a variety of fields. As a result, many extensions and modifications of the k-means algorithm have been suggested to eliminate shortcomings of the basic algorithm.

The k-means algorithm converges to a local optimum. Hence, the k-means algorithm does not necessarily generate optimal clusters. The clusters obtained by k-means may be very unbalanced. The quality of clusters produced by the

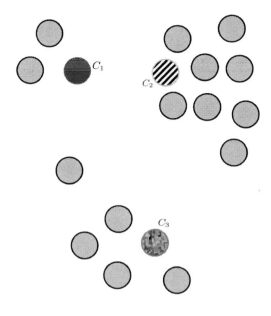

FIGURE 5.8: Initialisation of clusters

algorithm depends heavily on the initial choice of centres of clusters. It is also not obvious how to choose the magic number k. A modification to the basic algorithm, known as k-means++ [5], employs a smarter initialisation method and provides better clusters.

The process is sensitive to inputs which contain outliers. The algorithm is only useful for numerical attributes. The algorithm is not scalable. Bradley et al. [4] developed a scalable version of the k-means algorithm. But this algorithm stores the entire data in main memory. This algorithm, therefore, is not applicable for large datasets.

K-means clustering has been successfully applied to the domain of healthcare. It is seen that k-means help us to characterise subpopulations and diseases by medical conditions. Typical applications of the use of k-means are as follows:

1. Determining the group structure for diabetic/non-diabetic patients where ICD-10 code is not provided.

2. Grouping similar patients depending on features, such as cost, treatment, and outcome.

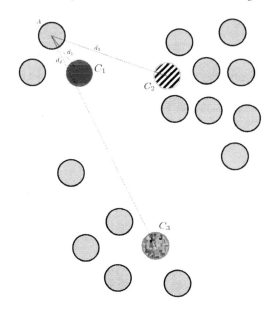

FIGURE 5.9: Assignment of points to clusters

5.4   Statistical Classifier: Bayesian and Naive Classification

A statistical classifier predicts the probability of an input belonging to a particular class. It is based on the Bayesian theory on conditional probabilities. It is one of the most-used approaches for certain types of learning because it is sometimes as good as decision trees and neural networks,

Classification by Bayesian networks uses the famous Bayes Theorem which is given in the following.

$$P(E|H) = P(H|E).P(E)/P(H)$$

$P(H)$ = Probability that a hypothesis H is true.
$P(E)$ = Probability that evidence E is true.
$P(H|E)$ = Probability that the hypothesis is true given the evidence.
$P(E|H)$ = Probability that the evidence is true given the hypothesis.

Let us take a small example. A laboratory performs a test say, T, which has only two outcomes: positive and negative. They guarantee that their test

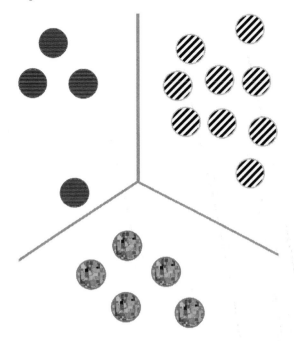

FIGURE 5.10: Assignment of points to clusters

result is 99% accurate. If 4% of all tests are actually positive and the test result is found to be positive, what is the probability that the test is actually positive?

Probability of a data actually being positive $P(T) = 0.04 = 4\%$.

Probability that data is positive given the laboratory result is positive $= P(C|T) = 0.99 = 99\%$.

Probability of data actually being negative $P(\neg T) - 0.96 - 96\%$.

Probability that laboratory gives positive result and the data is not actually positive $P(C|\neg T) = 0.01 = 1\%$.

$$P(C) = P(C|T) * P(T) + P(C|\neg T) * P(\neg T) = 0.0492$$

In order to calculate the probability that the data is actually positive given that the laboratory report says that the data is positive, that is $P(T|C)$, we will use Bayes theorem.

$$P(T|C) = 0.805$$

The naive bayes classifier [14], [16], uses the Bayes theorem. It computes the probability of data belonging to a specific class. The class with the highest probability is considered to be the most likely class to which the data belongs. This is also known as Maximum A Posteriori (MAP).

A priori probability $P(C|X)$ is the probability that an element belongs to the class C given the evidence X. This probability is calculated for each class and the class for which this probability is maximum is the desired class.

$$P(C|X_1, \cdots, X_n) = P(X_1|C) \cdots P(X_n|C).P(C)/P(X_1, X_2, \cdots X_n)$$

As $P(X_1, X_2, \cdots X_n)$ is the same for all classes, we ignore this quantity. And we maximize $P(X_1|C) \cdots P(X_n|C).P(C)/P(X_1, X_2, \cdots X_n)$ for each class C.

Suppose that we have a training dataset with 1500 records and 3 classes. The classes are: Sparrow, Fox, and Fish.

The Predictor features set includes Swim, Fly, Small, and Violent. All the features are either true or false.

Suppose that 50 out of 500 sparrows can swim. 450 out of 500 sparrows can fly. 450 out of 500 sparrows are small, and none of the sparrows are violent. 450 out of 500 foxes can swim. None of the foxes can fly, or are small. All foxes are violent. All fishes can swim. None of the fishes can fly. 100 out of 500 fishes are small, and 100 out of 500 fishes are violent.

Suppose that we have an animal which can swim, cannot fly, is small, and is not violent.

$$P(Fox|swim, small) = P(swim|Fox) * P(small|Fox) * P(Dog)/$$
$$P(swim, small) = 0.9 * 0 * 0.33/P(swim, small) = 0$$

$$P(Sparrow|swim, small) = P(swim|Sparrow) * P(small|Sparrow)$$
$$*P(Sparow)/P(swim, small) = 0.1 * 0.9 * 0.33/P(swim, small)$$
$$= 0.03/P(swim, small)$$

$$P(Fish|swim, small) = P(swim|Fish) * P(small|Fish) * P(Fish)/$$
$$P(Swim, small) = 1 * 0.2 * 0.33/P(swim, small) = 0.066/P(swim, small)$$

The value of $P(Fish|swim, small)$ is the greatest. Using naive Bayes, we predict that the data belongs to the class Fish.

5.4.1 Experiments with Medical Data

There are many medical problems in which the naive Bayesian Classifier has been used. A study in 2016 [16] reviewed published evidence about the application of naive Bayesian networks (NBN) in predicting disease, and showed that naive Bayesian networks perform better than many other algorithms. The authors studied 23 articles from PubMed published between 2005 and 2015 which covered about 53,725 patients for whom naive Bayesian network was applied for disease detection. The results obtained by naive Bayesian networks were better than those of many other algorithms. The metrics used were accuracy, sensitivity, specificity, and area under ROC curve. The illness covered in the 23 articles selected for the review included brain tumor, prostrate cancer, breast cancer, diabetic kidney disease, Type 2 diabetes etc. The results obtained by NBN is compared against neural network, logistic regression, SVM, decision tree, etc. The number of attributes chosen in these studies varies from four to several hundred.

In a frequently cited paper [14], the authors experimented with four medical problems: diagnoising the location of the primary tumour, predicting the recurrence of breast cancer, identifying diseases related to thyroid and rheumatology. The experiment was carried out using data at the University Medical Center in Ljubljana. The diagnostic problems are briefly described in the following.

- Localisation of primary tumour: The aim of the diagnosis is to detect the location of the primary tumour considering age, sex, the tissue pathology of carcinoma, the extent by which these tumours can be differentiated, and possible cites of metastases. Data of 339 patients was used in these experiments. For these patients, the location of the primary tumor was known. NBN was applied with 17 attributes.

- Prognostics of breast cancer recurrence: The aim of this task is to determine the probability of the recurrence of breast cancer within five years of surgery. The dependent factors include age of the patient, size of the tumour, its site and information about lymphatic nodes. The experiment used data of 288 patients. For these patients, whether recurrence of breast cancer within five years of surgery took place or not was known. Ten attributes were chosen.

- Thyroid diseases: The aim of this task is to determine one of four possible diagnoses about thyroid diseases. Dependent factors include age, sex of the patient, histological data, and outcomes of pathological tests. The experiment employed data of 884 patients whose final diagnoses were known. Fifteen attributes were considered.

- Rheumatology: The aim of this task is to chose one of six groups of possible diagnoses. The experiment employed data of 355 patients whose final diagnoses were known. 32 attributes were considered.

70% of instances were randomly used for learning and 30% percent were used randomly for testing in one run of the experiment. Ten such runs were carried out and average results were produced. A novel mechanism was employed to compare the accuracy of NBN with that of other methods. Four specialist doctors were chosen in each field. Random sample data from the training set were provided to them. For each patient, the doctors were asked to select the most probable diagnosis. The other conventional method employed was decision tree. NBN was seen to produce better results than an average physician or a decision tree.

5.4.2 Decision Trees

Classification of objects involves a set of training data where a number of objects and the classes to which these objects belong are known. Then, the problem is to compute the class given an object not present in the training dataset. Such a process of transforming findings from concrete examples (training data) to general models (process of inference) is called inductive inference. Instances are represented as a vector of attribute values. Learning an input implies that a set of instances and the classes to which these instances belong will be provided. The aim is to associate attribute values of instances to classes to which the instances belong. This association should be precise not only to classify training data but also to other unknown objects.

An overview of decision trees is presented in [19]. A decision tree [20] formalises building association between attribute values and classes. It consists of two categories of nodes: test or attribute nodes and decision nodes. Attribute nodes have two or more children, which are subtrees. Decision nodes are leaf nodes which are labeled with a class. A test or attribute node calculates certain outcome based on the values of the attributes of an object. Each outcome of the test in the test node is mapped to one of the children (subtrees) of that node. Classification of an instance starts at the root node. This node may be a test node or a decision node. If it is a test node, the outcome for the instance is computed and an appropriate subtree is chosen. The process continues from the root of the appropriate subtree. Finally, we encounter a decision node or a leaf node. Its label specifies the class of the object as predicted by the decision tree.

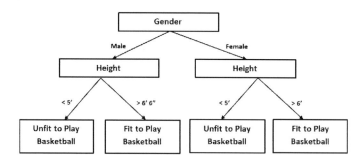

FIGURE 5.11: A part of a decision tree

First, the attributes of the dataset are chosen. Each attribute is associated with a class of values (value classes). If the values of an attribute are discrete, each value represents its own class; if the values of an attribute are continuous, some intervals are to be defined to represent different classes. An internal node in a decision tree corresponds to an attribute. The number of branches of an attribute node is the same as the number of distinct value classes that attribute has. The leaf nodes of a decision tree stand for the value classes of the attribute corresponding to a decision (Figure 5.11).

It is very easy to understand and interpret a decision tree. For example, see the part of a decision tree shown in Figure 5.11. Two rules can be inferred.

1. If the person is a girl and has a height of more than 6 feet, she is fit for playing basket ball.

2. If the person is a boy and has a height of more than 6 feet 6 inches, he is fit for playing basket ball.

A decision tree is built from a set of training data using a divide-and-conquer approach. There may be many attributes in a dataset. The question is which attribute to select for splitting. Suppose that we have a data of 30 persons. Each person is characterised by three attributes: sex (male/female), age (18/20), and height (5 to 6 ft). Twenty of them play football in their pastime. A decision tree is to be created to predict who will play football during leisure period. The root attribute will have to be the most significant input attribute out of three attributes, based on which maximum segregation of persons who play football in their pastime can be computed.

Many different algorithms are used in a decision tree to decide how to split a node into two or more sub-nodes. The idea is that the sub-nodes created will have increased homogeneity. The decision tree splits the nodes on all available attributes and then selects the split which results in the most homogeneous sub-nodes. GINI index of a node is computed based on different possible splitting. In the example, the root node may represent the attribute gender or class or height. Let us say, we take the root node for attribute gender. We compute the sub-nodes corresponding to male and female. Let us say that the proportion of football players in male is p and the proportion of football players in female is q. The GINI indices of the male team and female team are calculated as $p_1 = p^2 + (1-p)^2$ and $q_1 - q^2 + (1 \quad q)^2$, respectively. If the sizes of the male team and female team are m and n respectively, the GINI index at the root where the root corresponds to gender is computed as $m/(m+n) * p_1 + n/(m+n) * q_1$. Similarly, the GINI index is calculated for the root node corresponding to attribute age and attribute height. That attribute will be chosen as the root node whose GINI index is the highest.

Splitting can also be done on information gain. This criterion is based on an information theoretic term called Entropy. Entropy is the measure of degree of disorganisation in a set. If all the members of a dataset belong to the same class, the set is said to be pure and otherwise the set is said to be impure. Less information is needed to describe a pure class. So, its entropy is zero. Maximum entropy is set to 1. Entropy is calculated as per the following formula,

$$Entropy = -plog_2p - qlog_2q$$

where p and q are probability of success and failure. We calculate the entropy of the parent node and then the entropy of each individual node of the split, and calculate the weighted average of all the sub-nodes of the split. We take that attribute for splitting for which the weighted entropy of the subclasses is the minimum.

When all objects are of the same decision class (the value of the output attribute is the same), a tree consists of a single node, a leaf with the appropriate decision.

Decision trees are motivated by simple geometric concepts. Suppose that we have the following samples for two classes, represented by deep black and light black squares as shown in Figure 5.12. It is not possible to draw a single line of separation between these classes. We need two lines: one separating according to a threshold value of X and another according to a threshold value of Y as shown in Figure 5.13. The decision tree classifier repetitively divides the samples into subparts by identifying lines. It does so repetitively because there may be many distant regions of the same class divided by others.

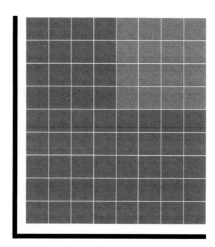

FIGURE 5.12: Samples of two classes that cannot be separated by a single straight line

5.4.3   Clasical Indction of Decision Trees

There are many specific decision-tree algorithms. The following algorithms are very popular.

In 1986, Quinlan introduced an algorithm ID3 (iterative dichotomiser 3) for generating a decision tree from a dataset [21]. Later, Quinlan developed an improved version of ID3 and named it C4.5. Other popular algorithms include

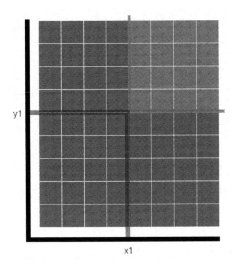

FIGURE 5.13: The sample separated by two lines

CART (classification and regression tree), CHAID (CHi-squared automatic interaction detector) and MARS.

The starting point of the ID3 algorithm is the original set S. This set is made the root node. The algorithm works on every unused attribute of S in each iteration. In every iteration, the entropy $H(S)$ or information gain $IG(S)$ of that attribute is calculated. The attribute with the minimum entropy (or the maximum information gain) is chosen and S is split using that attribute. The process is repeated on the generated subsets considering only attributes that were not selected before.

Suppose that $\{C_1, C_2, \cdots, C_k\}$ denote k classes, and T denotes a training set. The recursion stops under the following two conditions.

- If one or more objects belong to T, and all these objects belong to one class C_i, the decision tree is a leaf node representing the class C_i.

- If no object belongs to T, the decision tree is a leaf node using information other than T.

The ID3 algorithm can be summarised as follows:

- Compute the entropy of all attributes with the training data S.

- Select the attribute for which the entropy after splitting is the minimum or information gain after splitting is the maximum. Use this attribute to split the set S.

- Make a node in the decision tree for that attribute.

- Recursively apply the previous steps on subsets of S using the remaining attributes.

The following two metrics are used by the ID3 algorithm to facilitate splitting.

Entropy $H(S)$ of a dataset S is given by the following relation:

$$H(S) = \sum_{x \in X} -p(x) \log_2 p(x)$$

where $p(x)$ is the ratio of the number of elements in class x to the number of elements in set S and X is the set of classes in S.

Information gain $IG(A)$ is the measure of the difference between entropy of S before S is split and entropy after the set S is split, based on an attribute A. $IG(A)$ is expressed as follows:

$$IG(A, S) = H(S) - \sum_{t \in T} p(t) H(t)$$

T is the subsets created from splitting the set S on the basis of attribute A and $p(t)$ represents the proportion of the number of elements in class t to the number of elements in set S.

Quinlan went on to create another algorithm C4.5, which was an improved version of ID3. For example, C4.5 is able to take care of continuous as well as discrete attributes. Moreover, C4.5 can handle training data with missing attribute values by simply ignoring them in gain and entropy calculations. C4.5 can handle attributes which have different costs associated with them. C4.5 prunes the tree after creation. It revisits the tree after it is created and removes unuseful branches by replacing them with leaf nodes.

Advantages of using decision trees are as follows:

- It has already been pointed out that it is easy to understand and interpret decision trees.

- Numerical as well as categorical data can be handled by decision trees.

- Decision trees do not require much data preparations such as data normalization.

- Decision trees use a white box model.

- In decision trees, it is possible to validate a model using statistical tests.

- Decision trees represent human decision making more closely than other approaches.

- Decision trees can approximate any Boolean function.

But, they also have many limitations which are enumerated in the following:

- Decision trees may not be very accurate.

- Decision trees may not be robust. If the training data is changed in a small way, the decision tree may significantly change. This might lead to considerable changes in final predictions.

- The problem of creating an optimal decision tree even for simple ideas and for various aspects of optimality can be proved to be NP-complete. As a result, greedy algorithms and heuristics are used to generate practical decision trees. In such trees, approximate and not globally optimal decisions are made at each node. Such algorithms cannot guarantee to generate optimal decision trees. There are variants of decision trees to overcome some of these problems, such as the dual information distance (DID) trees.

- Decision trees may become excessively complex. This problem is also referred to as over-fitting.

- It is seen that information gain in decision trees has a bias towards attributes which have more levels.

5.5   Association Rule Mining (ARM)

We have already mentioned that today's healthcare industry produces huge amount of structured, semi-structured, and unstructured data. If this huge data can be used for knowledge extraction, it becomes immensely important. Such knowledge helps those in the healthcare field save costs and make effective decisions. Data mining techniques help us discovering hidden patterns, and knowledge from this huge amount of data.

There are several issues in using data mining tools for healthcare data. Sources of several data sets are various and this heterogeneity poses various challenges. Moreover, such data contains noise, outliers, and missing values. Transcriptions of patient records often have huge noise and a large number of missing values. Missing attribute values can affect the quality of analysis. At the preprocessing stage, data has to be cleaned and missing values have to be provided. Then, the right subset of data is to be chosen for successful data mining.

Data mining may be implemented for classification, clustering, and association rule mining. In this section, we have focused on the idea of association rule mining and its application in health data.

Classical association rules [28] are defined as in the following.

Let $D = \{t_1, t_2, \cdots t_n\}$ be a set of transactions in a database D. Let I be a set of items, $I = \{i_1, i_2, \cdots i_m\}$. The structure of an association rule is

$A \Rightarrow B$ (meaning A implies B), where $A, B \subset I$, and $A \cap B = \phi$. A is known as the left-hand side (LHS) or the antecedent of the rule. B is called the the right-hand side (RHS) or the consequent of the rule. A very common example of a rule applicable for data in a supermarket is $\{butter, bread\} \Rightarrow \{milk\}$. This implies that if a customer purchases butter and bread, he/she purchases milk, too.

In general, a set of items is called an itemset. For example, the antecedent and consequent of a rule is an itemset. There are many metrics associated with an itemset and a rule. The most common metric of an itemset is called support. This metric has statistical significance. For an itemset $A \subset I$, $support(A) = s$, is the fraction of transactions in the database containing items in A. One measure of strength associated with a rule is called confidence. It is defined as follows:

$$supp(A \Rightarrow B) = \frac{support(A \cup B)}{support(A)}$$

If the rule $\{butter, bread\} \Rightarrow \{milk\}$ has a confidence of 0.95, it implies that 95% of the time a customer purchases butter and bread, the customer buys milk well.

Discovering all the rules that have support and confidence greater than or equal to some thresholds which are already specified is known as the problem of association rule mining. To be statistically significant, a rule must have the support of several hundred transactions . Practical datasets typically contain thousands to millions of transactions.

There are many other measures of interest of rules such a lift and conviction.

$$lift(A \Rightarrow B) = \frac{support(A \cup B)}{support(A) \times support(B)}$$

If lift is greater than 1, it indicates the extent to which A and B are interdependent.

$$conv(A \Rightarrow B) = \frac{1 - support(A \cup B)}{1 - conf(A \Rightarrow B)}$$

5.5.1   Simple Approach for Rule Discovery

Many algorithms have been proposed for generating association rules. Apriori, Eclat, and FP-Growth are examples of a few such popular algorithms. However, these algorithms can only generate frequent itemsets. Generation of rules from frequent itemsets found in a database is the next step.

Apriori algorithm comprises two phases.

First Phase: All itemsets that have support greater than the threshhold are generated. These item sets are known as frequent itemsets. Other item sets are called infrequent. Itemsets having k elements are referred to as k-itemsets. First, all 1-itemsets are generated as candidates. Out of these candidates, itemstes which are found to be frequent according to their support are chosen to generate 2-itemssets. The same process is followed to generate 3-itetmsets. This process is continued. In this process, the number of items in itemsets is increased by one after each iteration. Also, transactions need to be scanned once in each iteration. This phase terminates when no frequent itemset can be found.

Second Phase: For each frequent itemset, all rules whose confidence is grater than a threshold are generated in the following manner. Consider any frequent itemset A and any $B \subset A$. If $support(A)/support(A \setminus B)$ is greater than the threshold, the rule $A \setminus B \Rightarrow B$ is selected as a valid rule.

5.5.2 Processing of Medical Data

An example of health data may be the profiles of patients in a hospital who are being treated for cardiac diseases [18]. Each record in such data contains relevant personal information of one patient such as age, race, smoker/non-smoker. Such data also contains medical information such as weight, heart rate, and blood pressure as well as pre-existing diseases and existing medical conditions. The diagnostics made by a physician are also contained in the record. All data are associated with time attributes. Then, all information related to tests and procedures that estimate the medical condition of the patient are also stored. Imaging information from various tests are also stored in the profiles of patients.

Before association rule mining (ARM) may be applied to such rich medical information, it needs to be converted into a transaction format. The medical data contains different types of attributes such as numerical, categorical, image, and time. To facilitate ARM, missing information has to be managed. A missing value may mean many different things. It may indicate that the person has no disease. In other cases, missing information may imply that this information is not applicable to the patient or simply that the information is not available. If association rules are mined using transactions with some records containing missing information in many fields, the rules so discovered may not be that reliable. It is not practical to discard records which have many missing values because that may reduce the available datasets to an unacceptable extent.

5.5.3 Association Rule Mining in Health Data

Association rule mining has been used to study the relationships among medical illness, lifestyles, and family medical history. Lifestyle variables include smoking, drinking, being overweight, etc. Medical illness may be hypertension, diabetes and similar such conditions. In a study of more than 5000 persons, more than 4000 rules were extracted.

Association rule mining has also been applied to brain tumour analysis breast cancer analysis, and oral cancer analysis. However, generation of knowledge in cardiac diseases has been more effective than that in tumour-related diseases.

ARM has been applied to bird flu, to explore epidemics such as dengue fever, and to study virus outbreaks such as, the Ebola virus with limited success. In case of such health crises, response has to be real-time. It may be noted that ARM application to these problems does not have acceptable response times.

5.5.4 Issues with Association Rule Mining

The major problems that are encountered while discovering interesting and reliable association rules in the medical domain are mentioned in the following.

Size of the association.
Association rules that contain a large number of items cannot easily be interpreted. So, the size of an association should not be larger than a given threshold. Most algorithms find all rules whose confidence is more than the minimum. In the medical domain that means generation of a huge amount of rules. The large size of the associations discovered slows down the algorithm considerably. Suppose that k-itemset X is frequent for a given support. Then all $Y \neq \phi$ and $Y \subset X$ are also frequent and this means that there are $O(2^k)$ frequent itemsets. It can easily be concluded that any algorithm, however efficient it may be, will become slow for large k. If $k > 8$, too many rules are produced rendering the results useless. Suppose that there are two rules $X_1 \Rightarrow Y$ and $X_2 \Rightarrow Y$ such that $X_1 \subset X_2$. Then, the
first rule is simpler and may have a larger support. If $Y_1 \subset Y_2$ and $X \Rightarrow Y_1$ and $X \Rightarrow Y_2$, the latter rule will probably have higher confidence but lower support.

Associations with uninteresting items.
Sometimes, certain itemsets are known to be trivial or have a very high support. In either case, such associations do not really reveal any new insight. Consider items i_j and $i_{j'}$. If the association $X_1 = \{i_j, i_{j'}\}$ does not bring out any new information, another association X_2 where $X_1 \subset X_2$ will not convey any new information either. Therefore, a domain expert may discard many such items as non-informative associations.

Performance of association rule mining.
Surprisingly, the Apriori algorithm is still used by health informatics research community to generate frequent itemsets in spite of the fact that the FP-Growth approach is more efficient. The Apriori algorithm is slower and less efficient than FP-Growth, especially for large-size databases.

Amount of data.

The efficacy of association rule mining depends on quantity, quality, and specificity of data. If the amount and variety of data is limited, the support of interesting association rules may be low or the level of belief may be weak. More data needs to be generated, which can significantly improve the results by increasing the support of interesting associations.

5.6 Time Series Analysis

A time series is a sequence of data measured normally over successive times. For example, the daily number of births or deaths, the number of admissions in a hospital, temperature readings at a place, expenditures over many years, or flow of a river are time series data. In time series forecasting, we first collect past observations and then these observations are analysed to create an appropriate mathematical model that implicitly contains the inherent process of data generation for the series. The events to take place in future can then be predicted using the model. The objectives of time series analysis include a simple description of the phenomenon, explanation of the phenomenon, prediction of future events, or control over the phenomenon. Such analysis is helpful in two cases: when sufficient knowledge about the statistical pattern of the observations is not available or when there is no appropriate explanatory model. In healthcare and biomedical research, the goal is to comprehend how explanatory variables influence an event over time. There is a difference between time series analysis and normal regression analysis. In normal regression analysis, the observations are assumed to be independent. In time series data, observations closer in time tend to be correlated with one another. In medical data, normal regression analysis is not valid as the observations are not independent. An example of time series data can be found in https://earthquake.usgs.gov. One example is shown in Figure 5.14.

A time series is non-deterministic in nature. So, it is not possible to forecast what will occur in future with absolute certainty . Therefore, we must take recourse to probability theory to analyse a time series. Generally, a time series is denoted by $\{x(t), t = 0, 1, 2, \cdots \}$ where each $x(i)$ represents a random variable. A stochastic process $\{Y_0, Y_1, Y_2, \cdots \}$ is a possibly infinite sequence of random variables ordered in time. So, a time series can essentially be viewed as a stochastic process. The sequence of observations of the series is nothing but one particular realisation of the stochastic process that produced it. In the context of a stochastic process, one interesting problem is to find the joint probability distribution of its random variables. An usual assumption in a stochastic process is that the random variables are independent and identically distributed (iid). However, observations in a time series analysis are not iids. For example, the temperature of a city on a day is not independent of

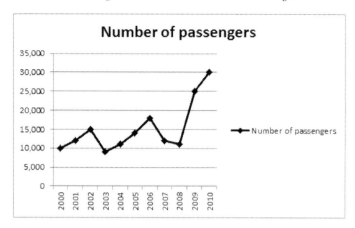

FIGURE 5.14: Annual number of passengers in an airline

the temperature of that city on the previous day. These considerations make time series predictions close to reality.

There are two related concepts in statistics which are useful in time series analysis: stationarity and ergodicity. If the joint probability distribution of the random variables at a time $(t_1, t_2, \cdots, t_n)$ is the same as the distribution of the variables at the times $(t_1 + \tau, t_2 + \tau, \cdots, t_n + \tau)$, the stochastic process is called stationary. The property of stationarity implies that the probability distribution of the set of random variables is independent of absolute times and does only depend on their relative times. In such time series, statistical properties such as mean, variance, autocorrelation, etc. remain fixed over time.

The ability to make valid probability statements by looking over time rather than across replicates at one time is called ergodicity.

5.6.1   Time Series Regression Models

When the objective of time series analysis is explanation, we model two time series: a response process $Y(t)$ and a predictor process $X(t)$. For example, suppose that we are interested in finding how deficiency in vitamin A, (X), affects the risk of acute respiratory infection, (Y). The objective is to determine the inter-dependency between vitamin A deficiency of children and the risk of acute respiratory infection (ARI). As Y is time series data, its neighbouring values will also tend to be correlated. The response process and the predictor process may be independent or dependent on each other. In this example, scientists report that acute respiratory infection may lead to loss of vitamin A and can lead to further deficiency. So, vitamin A deficiency and ARI processes are not independent. As Y_t is dependent on the past observations $Y_{t-1}, Y_{t-2}, \cdots, Y_1$ may be predicted from Y time series alone. Again, as

Y and X are interdependent, Y may be predicted using the covariate series X_t. When a value in a time series can be obtained from previous values of the same time series, it is called an autoregressive (AR) model. Distributed lag models are used to handle cases when a value in a time series cannot be obtained from previous values of the same time series.

Time series models may be linear and non-linear. Two widely used linear time series models are the autoregressive (AR) and moving average (MA) models. Autoregressive moving average (ARMA) and autoregressive integrated moving average (ARIMA) models are combinations of AR and MA models. ARMA and ARIMA models are derived from autoregressive fractionally integrated moving average (ARFIMA) models. The seasonal autoregressive integrated moving average (SARIMA) model, a variation of ARIMA, is used for seasonal time series forecasting. The famous Box-Jenkins principle is the basis of the ARIMA model and all its variants. So, these models are known as the Box-Jenkins models.

Linear models are relatively simple and easy to understand and implement. So, linear models are easy to describe. But non-linear patterns are embedded in many practical situations. Some non-linear models are: autoregressive conditional heteroskedasticity (ARCH) model and its variations, the threshold autoregressive (TAR) model, the nonlinear autoregressive (NAR) model, the nonlinear moving average (NMA) model, etc.

In this section, we shall discuss some important linear autoreagreesive time series models.

5.6.2 Linear AR Time Series Models

AR(p) and MA(q) models are combined suitably to develop ARMA(p, q) model. ARMA(p,q) is an effective mathematical tool to model a univariate time series. In an AR(p) model, the future value of a variable is estimated by a linear combination of past p observations, a random error, and a constant term. The AR(p) model can be mathematically expressed as in the following:

$$y_t = c + \sum_{i=1}^{p} \varphi_i y_{t-i} + \epsilon$$

Here, y_t represents the actual value at time t; ϵ represents random error; φ_i are model parameters, and c is a constant. p is an integer literal, which is called the order of the model.

MA(q) model uses past errors to predict the future value of a variable. The MA(q) model is expressed as the following equation:

$$y_t = \mu + \sum_{i=1}^{p} \theta_{t-i} \epsilon_{t-i} + \epsilon_t$$

Here, μ is the mean of the series; θ is the model parameter; q is an integer constant, which is called the order of the model. The random errors are assumed to be a sequence of independent and identically distributed random variables with zero mean and a constant variance σ^2. These are also called white noises. Generally, the random errors follow the normal distribution.

As we have already stated, ARMA(p,q) model is a combination of Autoregressive (AR) and moving average (MA) models. Mathematically, an ARMA(p, q) model is represented as follows:

$$y_t = c + \sum_{i=1}^{p} \varphi_i y_{t-i} + \sum_{j=1}^{q} \theta_j \epsilon_{t-j} + \epsilon_t$$

Lag operator notation can also be used to express ARMA models. Lag operators are also called backshift operators. They can be mathematically expressed as $L y_t = y_{t-1}$. ARMA models can be represented in terms of Lag polynomials as shown in the following.

Lag operator notation used to express AR(p) model as shown in the following:

$$\epsilon_t = \varphi(L) y_t$$

$$\varphi(L) = 1 - \sum_{i=1}^{p} \varphi_i L^i$$

Similarly, MA(q) model can be expressed in terms of Lag operators as shown in the following:

$$y_t = \theta(L) \epsilon_t$$

where

$$\theta(L) = 1 + \sum_{i=1}^{q} \theta_i L^i$$

ARMA(p, q) model expressed in terms of Lag operators:

$$\varphi(L) y_t = \theta(L) \epsilon_t$$

Stationarity Analysis

When an AR(p) model is represented by $\epsilon_t = \varphi(L) y_t$, $\varphi(L) = 0$ is known as the characteristic equation of the model. Box and Jenkins proved that an AR(p) process is stationary if and only if all the roots of the characteristic equation fall outside the unit circle. The conditions of ARMA model to be stationary and invertible are the same as those of AR and MA models. Thus, if all the roots of the characteristic equation $\varphi(L) = 0$ lie outside the unit circle, ARMA(p, q) process is stationary. Similarly, ARMA(p, q) process is invertible, if all the roots of the lag equation $\theta(L) = 0$ lie outside the unit circle.

Autocorrelation and Partial Autocorrelation Functions (ACF and PACF)

ACF and PACF analyses are carried out to find out a proper model for a given time series data. The coefficient of correlation between two values in a time series is called the autocorrelation function (ACF). The ACF for a time series y_t is given by the following equation:

$$Corr(y_t, y_{t-k})$$

k denotes the time gap between two values of a time series data. k is also called the lag. If lag is 1 in ACF, it denotes the correlation between values that are separated by one time unit.

The ACF attempts to measure the linear relationship between an observation at time t and observations taken at earlier times. If an AR(k) model is assumed, we would like to measure the relationship between y_t and y_{t-k} and ignore the linear influence of the variables that are between y_t and y_{t-k}. ACF cannot express such a relationship. In order to measure such a relationship, we require to transform the time series. Partial autocorrelation function (PACF) provides us the correlation of the transformed time series. The PACF is used to find out the order of an autoregressive model.

For covariate time series analysis, there are primarily two types of models: marginal and conditional [15]. The primary target of a marginal model is the expectation of Y_t. We do not compute Y_t using past responses $Y_{t-1}, Y_{t-2}, \cdots, Y_1$ as observations in a time series are autocorrelated. Rather, the correlation between all pairs of observations are modeled together. Therefore, the model comprises two components. First model is the normal regression model for the mean which is typical in cases of independent observations. The second one is for the autocorrelation function.

A simple marginal linear model is expressed by the following equations:

$$E(Y_t) = X_t \beta$$

$$Cov(Y_t, Y_{t-u}) = \sigma^2 \rho^u$$

Covariance among pairs of values which are separated by u time units is assumed to decrease exponentially with u. ρ denotes the correlation of two successive values which are separated by one time unit. This particular autocorrelation function is for a first-order autoregression model because this set of data is produced using the following equations.

$$Y_t = X_t \beta + \epsilon_t$$

$$\epsilon_t = \rho \epsilon_{t-1} + a_t$$

where a_t is white noise time series comprising independent observations with mean 0 and common variance $\sigma^2/(1 - \rho^2)$.

Alternatively, we can also model the conditional expectation of the response variable as a function of X_t and the past observations of the same time series $Y_{t-1}, Y_{t-2}, \cdots, Y_1$. For linear regression, a basic conditional model can be expressed as follows.

$$Y_t = X_t\beta + \alpha_1 Y_{t-1} + \cdots + \alpha_p Y_{t-p} + a_t$$

a_t is assumed to have independent and identical distribution with mean zero and a common variance.

Another alternative parameterisation of the previous model can be expressed as follows:

$$Y_t = X_t\beta + \alpha_1(Y_{t-1} - X_{t-1}\beta) + \cdots + \alpha_p(Y_{t-p} - X_{t-p}\beta) + a_t$$

In this formulation, the response is expressed based on deviation of previous response observations from their average and not on the previous observations themselves.

In that case, the marginal expectation is given by the following equation:

$$E(Y_t|X_t) = X_t\beta$$

5.6.3   Application of Time Series

DiPietro and colleagues [9] measured heart rate and movement of the foetus five times a second for a fifty-minute period. In this manner, they observed 120 mother-fetal pairs at 20, 24, 28, 32, 36, and 38-39 weeks of gestation. This is a multivariate time series where Y_t is a vector having two items Y_1 for fetal heart rate and Y_2 for fetal movement. Authors have also monitored mother's cardiac rate and skin conductance. They tried to figure out evolving interaction between mother and child in a quantitative manner through cross-correlation functions.

Overcrowding in hospital emegency department reduces quality of medical services. If monthly demand can be predicted, this problem may be solved in a better way. In [11], the authors attempted to predict the number of people visiting emergency department at a hospital in Taiwan by applying time series modeling and analysis. Specifically, they used ARIMA on data of the number of visits from 2009 to 2016.

Another instance of using time series modeling can be found in [6]. The authors have analysed the data of acute childhood lymphoid leukemia among Hungarian children using a seasonal time series model. They have also used ARIMA to study the Hungarian mortality rate.

5.7   Text Mining

T ext contains a huge quantity of qualitative information that is difficult to use in any kind of mathematical modeling. Text mining attempts to transform unstructured textual information into such meaningful numeric artefacts and sets of features so that data mining and machine learning algorithms can be applied on the extracted features. Thus, application of text mining is manifold, as will be discussed latter. Various tools and techniques used in text mining include term frequency, inverse data frequency, topic modeling, named entity recognition, sentiment analysis, to name a few. Using these tools and techniques, we can extract the necessary information and discover knowledge from textual information. Such knowledge discovery helps in getting effective insights, and finding out trends and patterns in huge volumes of unstructured text.

Typical Applications for Text Mining
Text mining has become immensely significant in recent times. Some of the application areas of text mining are listed below.

- Knowledge management: There is a huge amount of research data in fields like genomics and molecular techniques. There are volumes of clinical patient data. Text mining techniques are used to create knowledge management software that helps us in this direction.

- Spam filtering: Text mining techniques can effectively enhance the capabilities of spam filtering techniques which are based on statistics.

- Cyber crime prevention: Text mining intelligence adds power to anti-crime applications which may be used by law enforcement or intelligence agencies. Text mining technologies can also be combined with structured data. This technique is used by insurance companies to prevent fraud and process claims efficiently.

- Contextual advertising: Text mining can discover the subjective information from tweets, Facebook status, etc., which can be used for targeted advertising and customer care.

- Business intelligence: Text mining tools can ingest multiple data sources in real time. Such accurate semantic understanding with other artificial intelligence techniques helps large companies in decision making.

- Analysis of unstructured responses in surveys: In many surveys, there are certain open-ended questions where a person has to respond by providing subjective textual information. These questions are open-ended in the sense that the respondents are not constrained by any particular format or pre-specified set of responses. These allow the respondents to express their views. As an example, the respondents may be asked to write about advantages and disadvantages of using a product or service. It is possible to discover that the respondents are using a common set of words to express their views. By analysing these responses, insights into respondents' views and opinions may be discovered.

A brief overview of applications of text mining in healthcare data can be found in [22].

5.7.1   Term Frequency and Inverse Document Frequency

Suppose that we want to rank the relevance of a document based on some query containing a few words. We first eliminate documents that do not contain the words in the query. We can find out the frequency of occurrence of the words (terms) in these documents. We have to normalise this frequency considering many factors such as the size of the document. Thus, term frequency refers to the weight of a term that occurs in a document. Term frequency was introduced in 1957 by Hans Peter Luhn.

Various transformations of the frequency counts of words can be performed. Term frequency is not computed by raw number of occurrences of words. Term frequency is supposed to show how important a word is in a document. The importance of a word is not necessarily determined by its number of occurrences. For example, if a word occurs once in document A, but twice in document B, it cannot be concluded that this word is twice as important in B compared to A. So, a common way to measure term frequency , tf, of a word which occurs wf times in a document by the following formula:

$$tf(wf) = 1 + log(wf), \textbf{for } wf > 0$$

Sometimes, an even simpler transformation is used to measure term frequency.

$$tf(wf) = 1, \textbf{for } wf > 0$$

All terms in a query are not equally critical semantically. For example, the words like the, a, etc., in a query should be given less weight than more semantically rich terms to rank relevance of pages. So, inverse document frequency was introduced to measure the specificity of a term. The specificity of a term is inversely proportional to the number of pages in which it occurs. Inverse document frequency was introduced by Karn Sparck Jones in 1972.

$$idf(i,j) = \begin{cases} 0 & \text{if } wf_{ij} = 0 \\ (1 + log(wf_{ij}))log\frac{N}{df_i} & \text{if } wf_{ij} \geq 1 \end{cases}$$

In this formula, N is the total number of documents, and df_i denotes the number of documents that contain the i-th word. In other words, df_i is the document frequency for the i-th word. It may be observed that this formula absorbs two important factors. First, the log function causes a dampening effect for simple word frequencies. Second, it contains a weight factor that becomes zero when all documents contain a particular word. The same weight attains the maximum value if a word is contained in only one document. Thus, this metric reflects the relative frequencies of occurrences of words on one hand

and semantic specificity of these words in the set of documents on the other hand.

TF-IDF can also be used to classify documents and for prediction. For example, if we have 10 years of transcripts of calls by customers of a company, we may be able to classify them as calls by customers about to leave or calls by customers who want to complain, and so on. The matrix we mentioned earlier may be used as input to machine learning algorithms for such classification and prediction.

To facilitate TF-IDF computation and for many other applications, all words occurring in a corpus of documents may be indexed and counted. So, a matrix is created that specifies the number of times each word occurs in each document. In natural language processing, a corpus is usually described as a *BoW* matrix in which rows correspond to words and columns correspond to documents. The entries denote number of times a word occurs in a document.

5.7.2   Topic Modeling

A topic model discovers abstract topics occurring in a collection of documents. It is a probabilistic model. It is a powerful text mining tool that finds out dominant themes of a document. But besides text mining, it has applications in several other fields including computer vision, social networks, bio-informatics, etc.

A topic is regarded as a probability distribution over a fixed vocabulary. For example, suppose that there are three topics: protein, cancer, and computation. Each topic has a set of words. The probabilities of each word in a topic are arranged in the order of decreasing values. A document is assumed to contain a number of topics. The primary objective is to discover two things: (i) distribution of topics over each document, and (ii) distribution of words over each topic.

There are two popular approaches to topic modeling: latent dirichlet allocation (LDA), and probabilistic latent semantic analysis (PLSA). Suppose that the label of a document, a topic, a word are denoted by D, Z, and W respectively. Further, the number of words in D is denoted by N_D. The probability of topic Z in the document D, and the probability of word W in topic Z are represented by $P(Z|D)$, and $P(W|Z)$ respectively. In PLSA, we select a topic from the distribution over topics $P(Z|D)$ at random. Then, we select a word from the corresponding distribution over the vocabulary $P(W|Z)$.

$P(Z|D)$ and $P(W|Z)$, two distributions used in LDA are assumed to follow multinomial distributions. Thus, the topic distributions in all documents have the same Dirichlet prior α. Similarly, the word distributions of topics have the same Dirichlet prior η. If α and η are known for the document D, θ_D of a multinomial distribution over K topics can be computed from Dirichlet distribution $Dir(\theta_D|\alpha)$. Similarly, for topic k, β_k of a multinomial distribution over V words can be constructed from Dirichlet distribution $Dir(\beta_k|\eta)$.

A survey on how topic modeling can be applied in bioinformatics can be found in [17].

Stanford Topic Modeling Toolbox, R package topic models, Mallet (UMass Amherst), Python package, etc. provide a handful of effective tools for topic modeling.

5.8 Chapter Notes

- In this chapter, we have discussed how the source of healthcare data is huge in volume and the data source is varied. Analysis of several data formats has become very important in recent years.

- There are several data analysis methods available which can be employed for analysis of medical data.

- We have discussed artificial neural networks, which are also called connectionist systems. ANNs have been successfully used for medical diagnosis since the 1990s. The model, structure, and basic algorithm of a back propagation network have been discussed.

- Clustering is introduced as an example of unsupervised learning. The basic k-means algorithm is described.

- Nave Bayesian network has been introduced as a statistical classifier. The basic approach has been explained and its usefulness in medical data analysis has been discussed.

- Association rule mining is discussed next. Several important terms and sketch of a classical algorithm have been touched upon.

- Time series analysis has been briefly described. Linear auto regressive models are explained.

- Text mining is introduced as an important method to discover knowledge from an enormous volume of text data generated in the medical domain. Some tools of text mining have been discussed.

Algorithm 1 Training algorithm of a BPN

1: Initialise the weights and α, the rate of learning.
2: **while** termination condition is false **do**
3:     **while** there is a pair of training data **do**   ▷ Feed forward phase
4:         Each input unit takes an input signal x_i and propagates it to the hidden unit for all $i = 1$ to n.
5:         Compute the net input at the hidden unit as follows:

$$Q_{nj} = b_{0j} + \sum_{1=1}^{n} x_i v_{ij} \; for \; j = 1 \; to \; p$$

        If the signal from the i-th unit of the input layer is connected to the the j-th unit of the hidden layer, v_{ij} is the weight of that connection.
6:         Calculate the net output using the following activation function:

$$Q_j = f(Q_{inj})$$

7:         Propagate these output signals of the hidden layer units to the output layer units.
8:         Compute the net input at the output layer as follows:

$$y_{ink} = b_{0k} + \sum_{1=1}^{p} Q_j w_{jk} k \; for \; k = 1 \; to \; m$$

        w_{jk} is the weight on the k-th unit of the output layer coming from the j-th unit of the hidden layer.
9:         Calculate the net output using the following activation function:

$$y_k = f(y_{ink})$$

10:         Compute the error-correcting term.

$$\delta_k = (t_k - y_k)f'(y_{ink})$$

11:         Update the weight and bias as follows:

$$\Delta v_{jk} = \alpha \delta_k Q_{ij}$$

$$\Delta b_{0k} = \alpha \delta_k$$

12:         Propagate δ_k to the hidden unit.
13:         Each hidden unit will be the sum of its delta inputs from the output units.

$$\delta_{inj} = \sum_{k=1}^{n} \delta_k w_{jk}$$

14:         Compute the error term.

$$\delta_j = \delta_{inj} f'(Q_{inj})$$

15:         Update the weight and bias.

$$\Delta w_{ij} = \alpha \delta_j x_i$$

$$\Delta b_{0j} = \alpha \delta_j$$

16:         The weight and bias of each output of the output layer are updated as follows:

$$v_{jk}(new) = v_{jk}(old) + \Delta v_{jk}$$

$$b_{0k}(new) = b_{0k}(old) + \Delta b_{0k}$$

17:         The weight and bias of each output of the hidden layer are updated as follows:

$$w_{ij}(new) = w_{ij}(old) + \Delta w_{ij}$$

$$b_{0j}(new) = b_{0j}(old) + \Delta b_{0j}$$

18:     **end while**
19:     Determine whether the stopping condition has been reached. Stopping condition may be that the desired output matches with the actual outputs or the number of epochs has been reached.
20: **end while**

References

[1] Kazuto Ashizawa, Takayuki Ishida, Heber MacMahon, Carl J.Vyborny, Shigehiko Katsuragawa, and Kunio Do. Artificial neural networks in chest radiography: Application to the differential diagnosis of interstitial lung disease. *Academic Radiology*, 6(1):2–9, 1999.

[2] Turgay Ayer, Qiushi Chen, , and Elizabeth S. Burnside. Artificial neural networks in mammography interpretation and diagnostic decision making. *Computational and Mathematical Methods in Medicine*, 2013, 2013.

[3] Ashwin Belle, Raghuram Thiagarajan, S. M. Reza Soroushmehr, Fatemeh Navidi, Daniel A. Beard, , and Kayvan Najarian. Big data analytics in healthcare. *BioMed Research International*, 2015, 2015.

[4] P.S. Bradley, Usama Fayyad, and Cory Reina. Scaling clustering algorithms to large databases. In *KDD'98 Proceedings of the Fourth International Conference on Knowledge Discovery and Data Mining*, pages 9 – 11, 1998.

[5] Arthur David and Sergei Vassilvitskii. k-means++: The advantages of careful seeding. In *Proccedings of ACM eighteenth annual ACM-SIAM symposium on Discrete algorithms*, pages 1027–1035, 2007.

[6] Mria FAZEKAS. Time series models in medical resarch. *Periodica Polytechnica SER EL Eng*, 49(3-4):175–181, 2005.

[7] Aizenberg I., Aizenberga N, and Hiltnerb J et al. Cellular neural networks and computational intelligence in medical image processing. *Image and Vision Computing*, 19(4):177 – 183, 2001.

[8] Aleksander I. and Morton H. *An Introduction to Neural Computing*. Chapman and Hall, 1990.

[9] DiPietro JA, Irizarry RA, Hawkins M, Costigan KA, and Pressman EK. Crosscorrelation of fetal and somatic activity as an indicator of antenatal neural development. *American Journal of Obstet. Gynecology*, 185:1421 – 1428, 2001.

[10] J. Jiang, P. Trundle, and J. Ren. Medical image analysis with artificial neural networks. *Computerized Medical Imaging and Graphics 34 (2010) 617631*, 34:617 – 631, 2010.

[11] Wang-Chuan Juang, Sin-Jhih Huang, Fong-Dee Huang, Pei-Wen Cheng, and Shue-Ren Wann. Application of time series analysis in modelling and forecasting emergency department visits in a medical centre in southern taiwan. *BMJ Open*, 7(11):1–7, 2017.

[12] Karthik Kalyan, Binal Jakhia, Ramachandra Dattatraya Lele, Mukund Joshi, and Abhay Chowdhary. Artificial neural network application in the diagnosis of disease conditions with liver ultrasound images. *Advances in Bioinformatics*, 2014, 2014.

[13] Tapas Kanungo, David M. Mount, Nathan S. Netanyahu, Christine D. Piatko, Ruth Silverman, and Angela Y. Wu. An efficient k-means clustering algorithm: Analysis and implementation. *IEEE TRANSACTIONS ON PATTERN ANALYSIS AND MACHINE INTELLIGENCE*, 24(7):881 – 892, 2002.

[14] Igor Kononenko. Inductive and bayesian learning in medical diagnosis. *Applied Artificial Intelligence*, 7(4):317 – 337, 1993.

[15] Zeger Scott L, Irizarry Rafael, and Peng Roger D. On time series analysis of public health and biomedical data. *Annual Review Public Health*, 27:57 – 79, 2006.

[16] Mostafa Langarizadeh and Fateme Moghbeli. Applying naive bayesian networks to disease prediction: a systematic review. *Acta Informatica Medica*, 24(5):364 – 369, 2016.

[17] Lin Liu, Lin Tang, Wen Dong, and Shaowen Yaoand Wei Zhou. An overview of topic modeling and its current applications in bioinformatics. *SpringerPlus*, 5(1):1–22, 2016.

[18] Carlos Ordonez, Cesar Santana, and Levien de Braal. Discovering interesting association rules in medical data. In *Proccedings of ACM SIGMOD Workshop on Research Issues on Data Mining and Knowledge Discovery*, pages 78–85, 2000.

[19] V. Podgorelec, P. Kokol, B. Stiglic, and I. Rozman. Decision trees: an overview and their use in medicine. *Journal of Medical Systems*, 26(5):445 – 463, 2002.

[20] J. Ross Quinlan. *C4.5: programs for machine learning*. Morgan Kaufmann Publishers Inc., 1993.

[21] J.R. QUINLAN. Induction of decision trees. *Machine Learning*, 1:81 – 106, 1986.

[22] Uzma Raja, Tara Mitchell, Timothy Day, and James Michael Hardin. Text mining in healthcare. applications and pportunities. *Journal of healthcare information management*, 22(3):52–57, 2008.

[23] SAgatonovic-Kustrin and R Beresford. Basic concepts of artificial neural network (ann) modeling and its application in pharmaceutical research. *Journal of Pharmaceutical and Biomedical Analysis*, 22(5):717–727, 2000.

[24] Zhenghao Shi, Lifeng He, Kenji Suzuki, Tsuyoshi Nakamura, , and Hidenori Itoh. Survey on neural networks used for medical image processing. *International Journal of Computer Science*, 3(1):86 – 100, 2009.

[25] Chang Shu and Donald H. Burn. Artificial neural network ensembles and their application in pooled flood frequency analysis. *Water Resources Research - An AGU Journal*, 2004.

[26] Tutorialspoint. Artificial neural network: Supervised learning. Website: `https://www.tutorialspoint.com/artificial_neural_network/` `artificial_neural_network_supervised_learning.htm`.

[27] Dongkuan Xu and Yingjie Tia. A comprehensive survey of clustering algorithms. *Annals of Data Science*, 2(2):165 – 193, 2015.

[28] Mingzhu Zhang and Changzheng He. Survey on association rules mining algorithms. *Lecture Notes in Electrical Engineering*, 56:111 – 118, 2010.

[29] Zhi-Hua Zhou, Jianxin Wu, and Wei Tang. Ensembling neural networks: Many could be better than all. *Artificial Intelligence*, 137(1-2):239–263, 2002.

6

Architecture and Computational Models for Big Data Processing

CONTENTS

6.1   Introduction 130
6.2   Performance Issues 130
6.3   Parallel Architecture 135
     6.3.1   Distributed Shared Memory 137
     6.3.2   Hierarchical Hybrid Architecture 138
     6.3.3   Cluster Computing 138
     6.3.4   Multicore Architecture 139
     6.3.5   GPU Computing 140
     6.3.6   Recent Advances in Computer Architecture 141
6.4   Exploiting Parallelism 142
6.5   MapReduce Overview 144
     6.5.1   MapReduce Programming Model 146
     6.5.2   MapReduce Framework Implementation 146
6.6   Hadoop 148
     6.6.1   Hadoop Architecture 149
     6.6.2   Resource Provisioning Framework 149
     6.6.3   Hadoop Distributed File System 151
     6.6.4   MapReduce Framework 152
     6.6.5   Hadoop Common 153
     6.6.6   Hadoop Performance 153
6.7   Hadoop Ecosystem 153
     6.7.1   Apache Spark 154
     6.7.2   Apache ZooKeeper 155
6.8   Streaming Data Processing 156
     6.8.1   Apache Flume 156
     6.8.2   Spark Streaming 158
     6.8.3   Amazon Kinesis Streaming Data Platform 159
6.9   Chapter Notes 159

6.1   Introduction

One important challenge of big data analysis is processing the data with high quality, with reduced computing time and cost. Thus, performance is a major issue for big data analysis. From the early days of computing, developers, hardware engineers, and performance engineers have always focused on performance improvement of the software and system. Initially, in the sequential computers, the target was to improve the processing speed and reduce the memory access times. Two approaches for improving the processing speed were considered — first, to increase the clock speed by introducing a new hardware design for the chipset, and second, by increasing the number of processors and dividing the task among the processors for parallel processing. A number of architectures, in particular parallel architectures with multiple processors, evolved during the four decades starting with the 1970s. Architectural improvements were also made in order to reduce memory access times — for example, introducing various levels of cache memory, and making most data access from cache memory or local memory, etc. In this millennium, however, the focus shifted to using the powerful computing architectures built using commodity off-the-shelf computers. Therefore, the last decade and the present decade have seen the evolution of various novel computing concepts, such as cluster computing, and utility computing based on grid and cloud. Among these, the contemporary industries widely accepted the idea of cloud computing. *Big data processing* is mostly performed on cloud.

With the beginning of cloud computing and the Internet-based computing era, the performance issues became more complicated as the new challenge of data transmission over an unreliable network had to be taken into account. These challenges combined with specific challenges of big data handling have posed several tasks in front of the performance engineers for looking for solutions. This chapter will discuss the performance issues in high performance computing. It will also describe the traditional parallel architectures and the new evolving architectures for big data processing.

6.2   Performance Issues

Pfister [11] once pointed out that there are three ways of improving performance: (a) work harder, (b) work smarter, and (c) get help. 'Work harder' implies using faster hardware, i.e., high performance processors, memory, or peripheral devices. One can 'work smarter' by using the resources efficiently, i.e. writing efficient algorithms, etc. 'Getting help' refers to the use of multiple computers to solve a task. Whatever the approach is, performance in the high performance computing world often defines the time required by a computer to complete a task, i.e., the task *execution time*. However, depending on the context, performance may also involve one or more of the following metrics:

- Response time: Response time is the total amount of time a computer takes to respond to a request for service. A service can be fetching a word from the memory, storing or retrieving data to or from the disk, responding to a complex database query, or loading a web page. Generally, the response time is the sum of the service time and wait time.

- Throughput or rate of processing work.

- Availability of the computing system or application.

- Data transmission time, i.e., the time required to transmit data (a digital bit stream) over a point-to-point or point-to-multipoint communication link.

Further, when parallel computing is exploited in high performance computing, new performance metrics are required. In parallel computing, three important metrics are *speedup*, *cost*, and *efficiency*.

Speedup is a measure of relative performance, i.e. how fast a task can be completed on a multiprocessor system in comparison with a single processor system.

> **Speedup** — A ratio of the *execution time using a single processor system* to the *execution time using a multiprocessor system with p processors*. Thus,
>
> $$Speedup = \frac{execution\ time\ on\ single\ processor}{execution\ time\ on\ p\ processors} = \frac{T_s}{T_p} \quad (6.1)$$

There are two approaches which are adopted by the performance engineers for measuring the execution time on a single processor. In one approach, it is the execution time of the best-known sequential algorithm on a single processor of the system which is being used for executing the task. In the second approach, it is the execution time of the parallel algorithm on a single processor of the same computer. The latter is known as *self-speedup*.

Speedup can be *linear* (Figure 6.1 (a)), if it increases linearly with p, i.e., speedup is always p. It is super-linear (Figure 6.1 (b)), if speedup is larger than p. Otherwise, speedup is sub-linear (Figure 6.1 (c)). Sub-linear speedup is the general scenario for most tasks, although super-linear speedups can be observed sometimes due to cache effect or inherent parallelism in the algorithms.

Cost in parallel computing is defined as the execution time on p processors multiplied with p. Thus,

$$Cost = T_p \times p \quad (6.2)$$

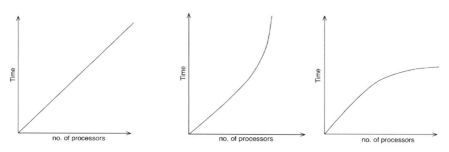

FIGURE 6.1: (a) Linear speedup, (b) Super-linear speedup, and (c) Sub-linear speedup

Cost may sometimes be referred to as the work done by the multiprocessor system.

Efficiency is measured to understand the effectiveness of parallel execution with respect to sequential execution. Thus, it is the ratio between the *execution time on one processor* and the *work done*. Thus, *efficiency* is defined as follows:

$$E = \frac{execution\ time\ on\ one\ processor}{execution\ time\ on\ p\ processors \times number\ of\ processors} = \frac{T_s}{T_p \times p}$$

(6.3)

A parallel program is work-optimal if efficiency is 1. Efficiency is sometimes expressed as a percentage; for example, efficiency of a computation may be 50%, which means that the processors are being used only half of their time for actual computation. The efficiency of 100% occurs when all the processors are used for the actual computation at all times and the speedup is p [17].

Scalability

Additionally, scalability is an important issue in parallel computing. Because in the case of multiprocessing systems, a task is divided into smaller pieces and distributed among the processors, one may think that if the number of processing elements is increased, the sub-tasks received by each processing element will be smaller and the execution time of the whole task will reduce. Thus, it may be believed that the larger the system, the better the performance at the time of execution. However, this is not the case.

One problem is that the number of processing elements and other units, like memory, peripherals, etc. cannot be increased indefinitely because of the limitation in the hardware design. Thus, *hardware scalability* or architectural scalability defines the enhancement in the size of the system (in terms of hardware resources, such as number of processors and memory) that can be achieved without compromising the system performance.

The other problem is to decide how far a task can be divided into smaller sub-tasks to execute on multiple processors and still continue to achieve speedup. It is noticed that due to several reasons, such as inherent characteristics of the algorithm, increase in the memory access and inter-processor communication costs, the speedup of a program may become saturated or deteriorate after certain increases in the number of processing elements. This situation actually hampers the performance of the program and is defined as the *algorithmic scalability*. Algorithmic scalability is important for big data analysis on today's computers.

Computation vs. Communication

As the sub-tasks have dependencies among themselves, processing elements may need to communicate. If they are connected with high-speed interconnection networks, as inside a multiprocessing server (a closely coupled system), the communication cost is very low and almost insignificant. However, the scalability of such systems is also low. On the other hand, processing elements may be connected using relatively low speed interconnection networks (as in the case of CPUs placed in a single box), or using local area networks (LAN) (as in the case of loosely-coupled computers connected as a cluster), or with a wide area network (WAN) or over the Internet (as in the case of grid or cloud computing). In all these cases, the communication cost increases depending on the speed of the network and the distances traversed by the pieces of data. A message passing programming paradigm is adopted by such systems where messages are passed between processing elements to transmit data and for synchronisation of the sub-tasks. Thus, here the execution time on p number of processors is denoted by

$$T_p = T_{comm} + T_{comp} \qquad (6.4)$$

where T_{comm} is the total communication time and T_{comp} is the computation time.

As the task is divided into smaller sub-tasks, the computation time generally decreases because the processing elements now need to do less work, whereas the communication time generally increases as more processes now communicate. This increases the amount of data transmission within the system and also the waiting time of the processes before receiving the necessary data to start or continue computation.

The communication cost is not present in sequential execution of tasks, and is therefore referred to as overhead. As long as the computation cost dominates the communication cost, performance improves. At some point of time, it may happen that the communication cost dominates; then the execution performance of the task degrades. The following metric is used to describe the effect of communication on the execution of tasks.

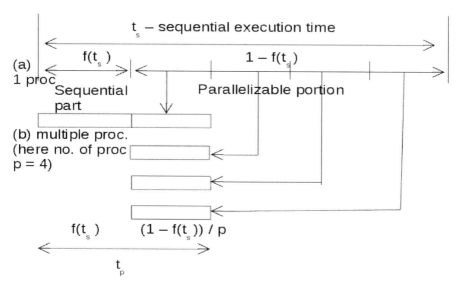

FIGURE 6.2: Execution of a parallel code - Amdahl's law

$$Computation/communication\ Ratio = \frac{Computation\ time}{Communication\ time} = \frac{t_{comp}}{t_{comm}}$$
$$(6.5)$$

The larger the ratio, the better the execution performance of the task.

Amdahl's Law

The question is how much maximum speedup can be achieved. There is always a portion of a program which cannot be executed parallely. This part of the computation cannot be divided into concurrent processes and must be executed serially. Thus, this part of the computation always limits the speedup. This situation can be expressed using the famous *Amdahl's law* [1]. If the fraction of computation which is to be performed serially is f, then the *speedup* factor on p processors is given by:

$$S_p = \frac{t_s}{f.t_s + (1-f)\frac{t_s}{t_p}} = \frac{p}{1 + (p-1)f} \qquad (6.6)$$

The time to perform the computation with p processors is given by $f.t_s + (1-f)\frac{t_s}{t_p}$. This is explained in Figure 6.2.

Other than communication overhead as explained in the previous section, several other factors may be present as overhead during the execution of a parallel program, and these factors limit the speedup which could be achieved by executing the parallel sub-tasks. The factors include (i) *time required for synchronizing the parallel parts*, (ii) *time spent for keeping processors idle due to non-uniform sized sub-tasks*, (iii) *the time needed to run an algorithm for scheduling and distributing the parallel tasks onto processors*, etc.

Moreover, it may be noted that a parallel execution may need to perform additional computation in comparison with sequential execution. For example, while computing the local variables within every parallel sub-task, additional computations are needed. Time is also required for additional 'load' and 'store' operations of the shared variables etc.

Such additional overheads also limit the speedup.

6.3   Parallel Architecture

Flynn's classification of computing architecture proposed in 1966 presented only four categories - 1) *Single Instruction Stream, Single Data Stream* (SISD), 2) *Multiple Instruction Stream, Single Data Stream* (MISD), 3) *Single Instruction Stream, Multiple Data Stream* (SIMD), and 4) *Multiple Instruction Stream, Multiple Data Stream* (MIMD). However, this taxonomy is too simple to describe the complex nature of the parallel hardware developed later.

The initial days of parallel computing have witnessed several dedicated parallel architectures which were introduced in the marketplace only for a few days and vanished thereafter without leaving any successors. At a later stage, mainly two architectural categories became stable — one is a single computer with multiple internal processors and a shared global memory, and the other is composed of multiple computers interconnected to form a coherent high-performance computing platform. These two basic types of parallel architectures are:

1. Shared Memory Multiprocessor

2. Distributed Memory Multicomputer

In general cases, a shared memory multiprocessor system is a natural extension of the single-processor machine. From the users' point of view, it is an extension of *von Neumann architecture*, in which multiple processors are connected to multiple memory modules through an *interconnection network* as shown in Figure 6.3. The memory modules are shared among the processors, which means that any processor can access any location in the memory modules using simple memory 'load' and 'store' primitives. In this architecture, each processor uses the shared bus to access the memory, and the access time is independent of the data location within the memory. Therefore, memory access time is uniform across all processors and it also remains the same regardless of which memory location is accessed to retrieve the data. Thus, such

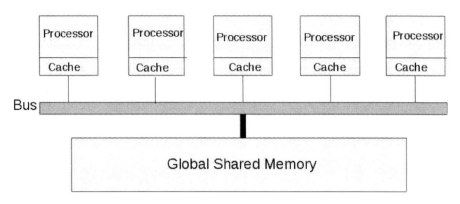

FIGURE 6.3: Shared memory multiprocessors

an architecture is also referred to as *Uniform Memory Access* machine, or UMA.

From a programmer's point of view, the shared memory multiprocessing systems are attractive because of the simplicity of the programming model used here. Typically, the executable code and all data are stored in the shared memory and all processors execute the same program. Thus, with respect to the programming model, it is similar to Flynn's category of *SIMD* machine.

However, due to physical limitations of the bus or other types of interconnection networks, the scalability is an issue. It is not practical to build a large-scale shared memory machine with all processors having fast and uniform access to the entire memory. Although several two-processor or four-processor machines have been built around this architecture, building a real large-scale multiprocessing system is not possible.

Often, the processors in the shared memory machines come with additional cache memory. The cache memory is generally private to the respective processors. If caches on multiple processors store copies of the same data, consistency of data needs to be maintained by using a special hardware design.

An alternative to the UMA machines is an architecture based on multiple computers connected through an interconnection network as shown in Figure 6.4. Each computer consists of a processor and local memory. Any processor can access its own local memory for executable code and data. In order to access the remote memory modules, a processor needs special programming constructs. The message passing programming paradigm is generally used for such types of systems. A processor sends messages to other processors. The messages carry data from one processor to other processors as per the requirements of the program. Such multiprocessor systems are usually called *message-passing multiprocessors* or *multicomputers*. These multicomputers are easier to scale compared to shared memory multiprocessors. Therefore, large-scale systems can be built with this architecture.

There is no doubt that the scalability of such a distributed architecture is

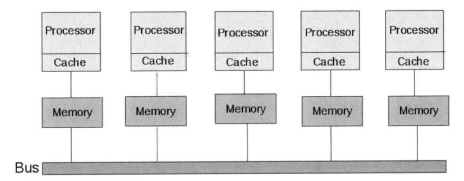

FIGURE 6.4: Distributed memory multicomputer

high. Due to the proximity of each processor to its own local memory, data locality can be exploited, thereby reducing the average memory access time. The architecture is also cost-effective as there is no need for using special hardware, and off-the-shelf commodity hardware can be used. In spite of the above benefits, the message passing programming paradigm requires the programmers' clear understanding about how a task (to be executed by a program) will be divided into different sub-tasks (to be executed by different processes running on multiple processors) to achieve maximum performance improvement. It also requires the programmers' knowledge about special programming constructs or *message passing libraries*, such as MPI.

6.3.1   Distributed Shared Memory

In order to make parallel programming easy, *distributed shared memory machines* have evolved that allowed the memory modules of multicomputers to be logically shared by all the processors. A memory mapping manager (usually a software module) of each node maps its local memory onto a virtual shared memory (Figure 6.5), thereby presenting a logical view of *shared address space*. The processors access their own local memory modules in less time. Accessing remote memory modules attached with other processors requires a longer time, but can be accessed using similar simple memory access constructs as used for accessing the local memory. Thus, the memory access time varies with the location of the data to be accessed. If data resides in local memory, access is fast. If data resides in remote memory, access is slower. As opposed to UMA, the term *Non-Uniform Memory Access* or NUMA is used for such types of architectures. The advantage of the NUMA architecture also lies in the fact that the average access time can be improved with the use of fast local memory and exploiting locality of data.

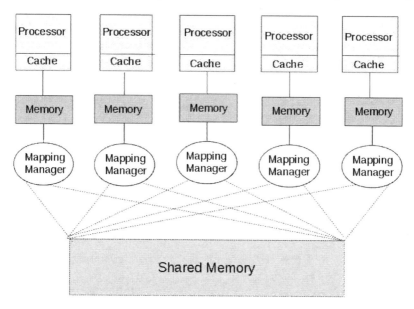

FIGURE 6.5: Distributed shared memory

6.3.2   Hierarchical Hybrid Architecture

Modern multiprocessor systems mix the above basic architectures. In the complex hierarchical scheme shown in Figure 6.6, processors are grouped by their physical locations on a specific node. Processors within a node share access to memory modules as per the UMA shared memory architecture. At the same time, they may also access memory from the remote nodes using a shared interconnect, but with slower performance as per the NUMA shared memory architecture.

6.3.3   Cluster Computing

Typically a cluster computer architecture is based on the multicomputer model. A group of computers, usually connected through a commodity network, and working together closely so that in many respects they present a *single system image* (SSI) view to the users, is called a cluster. The components of a cluster are commonly, but not always, connected through fast local area networks. Each computer runs an operating system and is also loaded with a cluster middleware which creates an integrated single system view for all the computers in the cluster. Generally, one of the computers or nodes plays the role of a master, whereas the others become the workers. The master computer divides a program or a task into small sub-tasks and sends a sub-task to each node for processing. When nodes finish their allotted tasks, the master computer sends more tasks to them until the entire problem is computed.

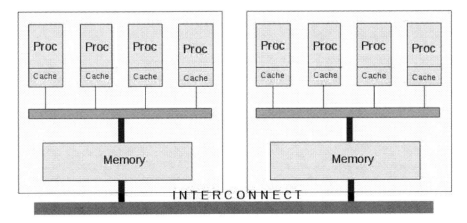

FIGURE 6.6: A hierarchical hybrid architecture

Other than improving the program performance through parallel processing, a cluster is also used for *high availability*, i.e., even if a node crashes or stops working, other nodes continue the processing of the program or task. *Beowulf cluster*, which is constructed from a collection of generic computers running commonly used operating systems (such as Linux) and connected through an interconnect (such as Ethernet), has become one of the most popularly used clusters worldwide because of its cost-effectiveness [14]. Parallel processing of tasks on such clusters can be availed with commonly used parallel processing libraries, such as Message Passing Interface (MPI) and Parallel Virtual Machine (PVM).

6.3.4 Multicore Architecture

Modern computers are based on multicore processors. A multicore processor is an integrated circuit in which two or more processing units are placed together to enhance performance and reduce power consumption. Different threads of execution can be allocated to different cores, thereby extending support for parallel processing within individual software applications. As cores are placed on an integrated chip, the distances between them become quite small. This reduces memory access latency and increases cache speeds when compared to using separate processors or computers. However, although caches at the nearest level of the cores may be non-shared, the cores on a single chip share some of the on-chip resources, such as L3 cache, system bus, memory controller, I/O controllers and interconnects, and also external resources, such as main memory, I/O devices and networks. Thus there are always chances of single points of failure. Moreover, two applications sharing the resources can interfere with each other, and can impact their performances. However, in the absence of suitable lightweight libraries for muticore architectures, the possibility of engaging multicore systems in large-scale parallel processing has not yet been widely explored.

6.3.5   GPU Computing

GPU computing is based on a model of using CPU and GPU (i.e., *Graphics Processing Unit*) together to build a heterogeneous computing model. Each application has a sequential part which either cannot be parallelised, or the overall performance degrades if the portion is parallelised, and therefore, this portion is run serially on a CPU. The computationally-intensive part is parallelised and executed on the GPU, so that the performance improves. Applications in the areas of deep learning, analytics, and engineering run much faster on a GPU.

For many years, GPUs have been used to accelerate the graphics pipeline. However, in the last decade, it was felt that they can be extensively used for data parallel applications for processing non-graphical entities. These GPUs used for general purpose computing are known as the General Purpose GPUs or GPGPU [1]. In contrast with CPUs, GPUs have many math units, fast access to onboard memory, and therefore, they are very efficient for data parallelism and applications with higher arithmetic intensity for parallel nature, such as floating point operations.

A GPU architecture is a massively parallel architecture based on Flynn's SIMD concept. the architecture generally comprises three basic parts as described in NVIDIAs GPU architecture CUDA (Compute Unified Device Architecture) [10]. The device is split into grids, blocks, and threads in a hierarchical structure, as shown in Figure 6.7. A grid contains several blocks and a block contains several threads. The device becomes able to achieve massive parallelism using such a hierarchical architecture.

CUDA architecture is built around a scalable array of multithreaded Streaming Multiprocessors (SMs) or grids. The SM contains a few scalar cores and clocks which can run simultaneously. Each core either executes identical instruction sets, or sleeps. Instructions are scheduled across cores by the SMs with 0 overhead. Many threads may be scheduled on a core at one time, called a warp, but a certain maximum number of warps are active in one SM. The numbers depend on the actual version of the device.

Figure 6.8 shows the memory model of CUDA architecture. It has a *global memory* for read and write operations which are performed at the grid level. It is slow and does not have any cache. Therefore, memory access pattern is important when using this memory. On the other hand, *texture memory* at grid level is read-only memory. Its cache is optimised for 2D spatial access patterns. There is another read-only memory at grid level, known as *constant*

---

[1]NVIDIA, a pioneer in GPU computing, first brought GPU accelerators to the market in 2007 for general purpose use. Within a few years, these GPU accelerators have become part of power energy-efficient data centers in government labs, universities, enterprises, and small-and-medium-sized businesses around the world.

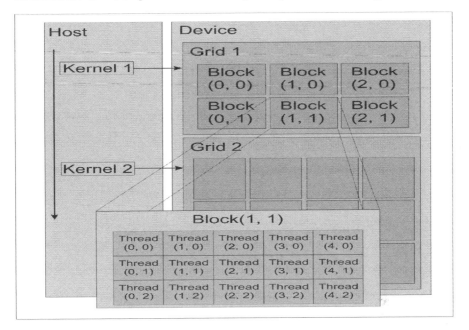

FIGURE 6.7: GPU architecture [Source: [10]]

memory. The constants and kernel arguments are stored in *constant memory*. It is slow, but contains cache. All threads in a block can use *shared memory* for read or write operations. It is shared among all threads in a block and its size is smaller than global memory. The number of threads that can be executed simultaneously in a block is determined by the shared memory that is specified, and it denotes the occupancy of that block. Thread-level memory sharing is supported via shared memory. There are two other memories which are local to each thread. *Register memory* is local to the thread, and is the fastest memory available in GPU architecture. Additionally, *local memory* is used for any data that does not fit in registers. Local memory is slow and does not have any cache, but allows automatic combined read and write operations. Figure 6.8 gives an overview of the memory model of GPU architecture.

6.3.6 Recent Advances in Computer Architecture

With the advent of web-based computing and mobile computing, energy usage and application performance are being considered as the primary issues in computing. Recent technological innovations, with specific focus on these two issues, are therefore causing a major change in computer hardware architecture [2]. The traditional way of thinking about computing on single or multiple hosts has been CPU-centric, where data is fetched from storage or memory, and moved closer to the CPU on which computation is performed.

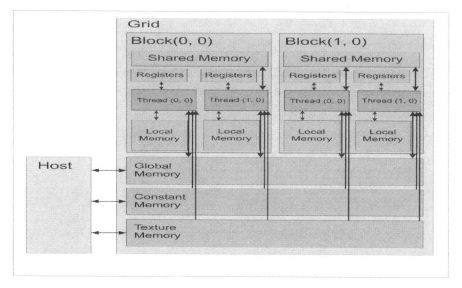

FIGURE 6.8: Memory organization in a GPU architecture [Source: [10]]

However, with the increased programmability offered by modern devices, such as *solid state drives* and *memory interfaces*, the traditional form of computing has changed. One important concept that evolved during the last two decades is *Near Data Processing* (NDP). In NDP, specific computations are brought near the data stored on storage devices and executed on the low power and low frequency cores in the storage devices [3]. A similar trend is observed in high performance computing for scientific or financial applications. The applications offload computations onto co-processors to exploit the high degree of parallel processing capabilities present in them.

6.4   Exploiting Parallelism

In order to exploit parallelism in a task, the programmer follows a parallel programming model, i.e., picks up a conceptualisation of the machine in abstract form for developing parallel applications. The most popular programming models or programming paradigms are:

- Multiprogramming model: A set of independent tasks, which do not require any communication or synchronisation at program level. Examples include a web server sending pages to browsers.

- Shared address space model: Tasks operate and communicate via shared data, like bulletin boards.

- Message passing programming: Explicit point-to-point communication is performed between the tasks running as different processes. It is analogous to phone calls (connection-oriented) or emails (connectionless, mailbox posts).

In a shared address space model, a process contains a virtual address space and one or more threads of control. Portions of the address spaces of the processes are shared among all processes. Hence, 'writes' to this shared space are visible to other threads within the same process or in other processes as well. This being a natural extension of the uniprocessor model, conventional memory 'read' and 'write' operations are used. Special atomic operations, such as locks, are implemented for synchronisation.

Some portion of the virtual address space is private to the process and only copies of the private variables are stored in these memory locations.

In contrast with the shared address space programming model, processes in the message passing model store and access data only in the local, private memory. The processes run independently and communicate with each other through explicit 'message passing' commands. Typically, a sending process issues a 'send' instruction to send data to another process and the receiving process issues a 'receive' instruction. When there is a match, then communication happens between the two processes.

While using either of the above-mentioned programming models, either a task-parallel or a data-parallel (or a hybrid) approach is followed to generate the parallelisable sub-tasks. In the case of a task-parallel approach, each processor is assigned with a different task, thereby functioning in an MIMD paradigm. In the shared address space programming model, this is implemented with a fork-join model [2] with thread-level parallelism, and communication is via the shared address space using memory read and write constructs (such as *memory load* and *memory store*). In the message passing model with distributed processing, task-parallelism is implemented with processes and communication is through explicit message passing (such as *send* and *receive*) among the processes. In both cases, synchronisation is explicit (via locks and barriers).

On the contrary, in case of a data-parallel approach, an SIMD paradigm is exploited. Multiple processors (or units) operate on segmented data sets. Tasks execute the same code and take identical actions on different parts of the data. Communication is done via shared memory or logically shared address space. Thus, on shared memory architectures, all tasks may have access to the same shared data structure through global memory. On the other hand, on distributed shared memory architectures, the data structure is split up and its parts are distributed as 'chunks' to reside in the local memory of each processor executing a parallel task. Synchronisation is implicit in this case. The data parallel model has the following characteristics:

- The parallel tasks focus on performing operations on a data set.

---

[2] A large task is divided into smaller sub-tasks and the sub-tasks are executed parallelly. Finally, the results are combined when execution of all the smaller tasks is completed.

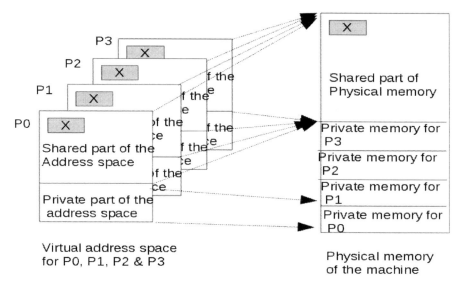

FIGURE 6.9: Shared Address Space programming model

- The data set is typically organised into a shared, common structure, such as an array or cube.

- A set of tasks work collectively on the same data structure; however, each task works on a different partition of the same data structure.

Data parallel operations are performed on shared data and private data is defined explicitly. Thus, data parallel approaches are suitable for exploiting parallelism in loops. On the other hand, in case of task parallelism, operations on private data are emphasised and explicit constructs are needed for sharing data and synchronisation.

A hybrid model combines the two previously described models. One example of a hybrid model is the combination of the message passing model with the threads model. Threads perform computationally intensive parallel tasks using locally stored data, and communications between processes on different nodes occur over the network using message passing constructs. Figure 6.9 and Figure 6.10 depict the shared address space programming model and the message passing programming model, respectively.

6.5   MapReduce Overview

MapReduce is a programming model originated from Google by Jeffrey Dean and Sanjay Ghemawat [6] [7]. The programming model was inspired by 'the

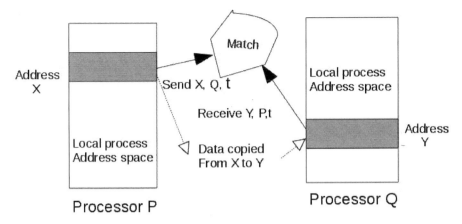

FIGURE 6.10: Message Passing programming model

map and reduce primitives' present in LISP and several other functional programming languages. In LISP, the map function takes a function and a set of values as parameters. That function is then applied to each of these values. The reduce function is given a binary function and a set of values as parameters. It combines all the values together using the binary function. It was observed by Dean and Ghemawat that most of the computations performed by applications usually involved a *map* operation to each logical record in the input in order to compute a set of immediate key/value pairs, and then a *reduce* operation to all the values that share the same key, in order to combine the derived data appropriately [6] [7]. They also pointed out that most such computations are conceptually straightforward. Nevertheless, the computations need to handle huge amount of input data involving several computational cycles. The computations can actually be distributed among many processors (or computers) to be executed parallelly and thus can be completed in a reasonable amount of time. In order to handle the distribution of computations across the computers, to execute them parallelly and to gather the results, to handle failures and for similar other tasks, the programmers need to write complex code that obscures the original simple computations. Hence, Dean and Ghemawat from Google started building a framework that abstracted all the common codes for parallel computing, and provided a set of APIs to the users to simplify the processing for the framework users. Users just need to write simple map and reduce functions. The Google MapReduce library was developed using C++. Later, the MapReduce idea was picked up by Yahoo as an open-source project and the framework, which got a new name, *Hadoop*, was developed in Java.

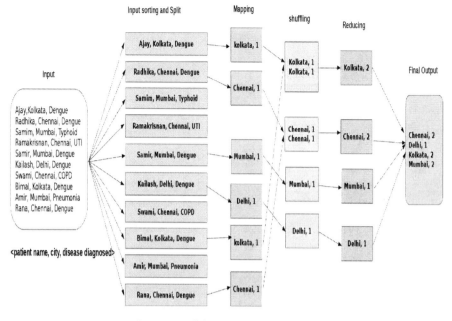

Query: count all dengue patient location wise

FIGURE 6.11: A workflow of MapReduce program

6.5.1   MapReduce Programming Model

The programming model primarily depends on the invocation of two functions, namely *map* and *reduce*. The *map* function reads a stream of data, parses it and produces a set of intermediate key/value pairs. All these values which are associated with the same intermediate key I are grouped together and passed to the *reduce* function. The *reduce* function accepts the intermediate key I and merges the set of values associated with the key to produce a single value or a smaller set of values. *Reduce* is invoked each time for a unique key. The keys are presented in sorted order. For example, while counting the access frequency to a URL, the map function parses logs of web page requests and outputs $(URL, 1)$. The reduce function adds together all values for the same URL and emits a $(URL, totalcount)$ pair [6] [7].

A workflow of MapReduce program for counting the number of 'dengue' patients in different cities is shown in 6.11.

6.5.2   MapReduce Framework Implementation

Dean and Ghemawat also pointed out that implementation of MapReduce should depend on the underlying execution environment. For example, frameworks targeting small-scale symmetric multiprocessors (SMPs) should be different from the frameworks targeting large-scale NUMA multiprocessor systems or those targeting larger collections of loosely-coupled networked computers. The initial framework originated by Google was targeted on large clusters of commodity PCs connected together with switched Ethernet [4].

The original MapReduce execution overview is shown in Figure 6.12 [6] [7]. The framework is based on a *single master and multiple workers* model. The workers may be assigned a *map* role or a *reduce* role. The execution of a MapReduce program is performed in the following steps:

- The input data is split into several pieces, known as **splits** or **shards**. The user program can specify the nature of these splits based on certain file formats.

- A single master and several worker processes are created as defined by the user. The master is responsible for dispatching the jobs to workers, keeping track of the progress of the workers, and returning the results.

- A number of *map workers* then read from the respective splits as assigned to them by the master. While parsing the pieces, they disregard the data which are of no interest and generate *key, value* pairs for the data of interest. The *key, value* pairs produced in this manner are buffered in the memory. All these are done parallely by the *map workers* executing on multiple computers in the network.

- The buffered *key, value* pairs are periodically written onto the local disk. While writing on the disk, a partitioning function partitions the buffered data into a number of regions. The locations of these regions are sent back to the master, who subsequently forwards the locations to the *reduce workers*.

- The *reduce workers*, after being notified by the master, read the buffered data from the local disks of the *map workers* using remote procedure calls. The data are then sorted by the *key* and all occurrences of the same key are grouped together.

- The *reduce workers* then invoke the *reduce* function which is defined by the user. Each worker passes the key and list of corresponding values to the *reduce* function. The output of the *reduce* function is appended to a final output file for the partition.

- After all the *map workers* and *reduce workers* complete their tasks, the result is returned to the user program by the master.

The MapReduce library proposed in [6] [7] also handles the fault tolerance issue. Since a huge volume of data is handled by the MapReduce execution environment and a large number of computers are involved, periodical checking of the functioning of the workers is required. The master therefore pings the workers regularly and whenever it does not get any response from a worker within the stipulated time, it considers the worker to have failed. The ongoing

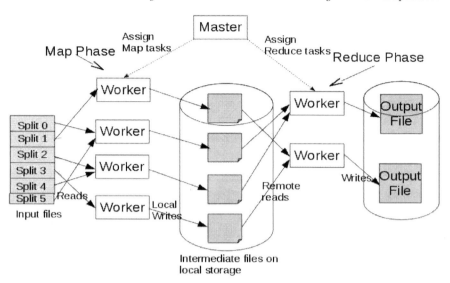

FIGURE 6.12: MapReduce execution environment [Source: [6] [7]]

task (a map task or a reduce task) on the failed worker is then returned to the initial state and is prepared for rescheduling. A completed map task on the failed worker needs to be redone as its results are stored only on the local memory of the worker. On the other hand, the completed reduce task does not need to be scheduled again as its results are stored in the global file system.

One important aspect of MapReduce programming is taking the piece of code near the data for execution. This saves the time required to transmit the voluminous data over the network for execution. Thus, in order to exploit the locality of data, the master in the MapReduce execution environment gathers location information about the data and attempts to schedule the map task on a machine that contains a replica of the corresponding input data.

After the initial implementation of the MapReduce execution environment by Google [18], it was picked up by Yahoo and re-implemented in Java as a open-source platform, called Hadoop. The Hadoop implementation is described in the following section.

6.6   Hadoop

Hadoop is an open-source framework based on the MapReduce programming model. Hadoop facilitates storage of voluminous data in a distributed environment across clusters of computers and processing of this data using simple programming models. It is designed to scale up from a single server to thou-

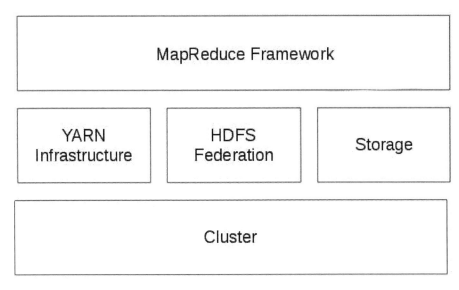

FIGURE 6.13: Hadoop architecture overview

sands of machines, each executing the task independently and offering local computation and storage.

6.6.1 Hadoop Architecture

At the bottom layer of the Hadoop architecture lies a cluster of networked computers or **nodes**. Nodes are sometimes partitioned into **racks**. On top of this layer, there are the following components: i) a framework for provisioning the computational resources, ii) a framework for providing permanent, reliable, and distributed storage, and iii) additional storage solutions.

Hadoop YARN is responsible for provisioning computational resources, i.e., resource management and scheduling. Many application frameworks can be implemented on top of YARN framework. Presently, only a MapReduce-based framework is implemented. Figure 6.13 shows an overview of Hadoop architecture [5].

6.6.2 Resource Provisioning Framework

The *resource provisioning framework* in Hadoop, the *YARN Infrastructure* (Yet Another Resource Negotiator), handles computational resources, i.e., CPUs, memory, etc. It has one **ResourceManager** component and several **NodeManager** components.

The ResourceManager, which plays the role of a master, keeps track of the locations of the NodeManagers and their resources. It also offers various services. The most important service is the *resource scheduling* service. Other

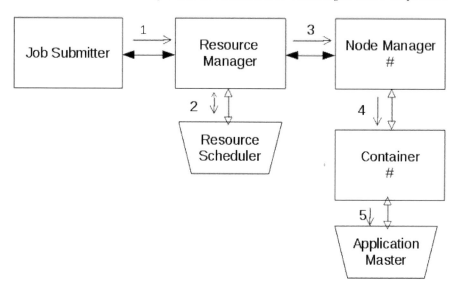

FIGURE 6.14: YARN application execution

services include monitoring the liveness of the application, and monitoring the liveness of the node managers and various event handlers.

There may be many NodeManagers in a cluster. The NodeManagers are the workers and each NodeManager carries the responsibilities of managing the resources on a particular node or rack. Its resource capacity is defined by the number of vcores (or virtual cores)[3] and the amount of memory. At the time of execution, the ResourceManager decides how much of these resources will be used by the user program and accordingly creates a **container**, which constitutes of a fraction of the NodeManager's resources. Thus, a NodeManager offers resources to multiple containers.

Within the YARN framework, many actors assist to execute a client job. At the beginning, the **job submitter** (i.e., the client) submits an application to the ResourceManager. The ResourceManager, with the help of the **resource scheduler**, allocates a **container** for the job. It also contacts the related NodeManager. In response, the NodeManager launches the container and the **ApplicationMaster** is placed on the container for execution. The ApplicationMaster negotiates for resources with the ResourceManager and provides framework-specific libraries to support the NodeManager(s) in executing the tasks and monitoring their executions. Figure 6.14 depicts the execution of an application on top of YARN.

---

[3]'Virtual cores' are merely abstractions of actual cores. The abstraction allows YARN to dynamically spin threads based on availability.

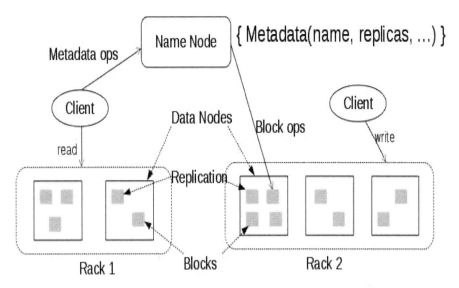

FIGURE 6.15: HDFS architecture

6.6.3 Hadoop Distributed File System

The Hadoop Distributed File System (HDFS) is the main storage system used by applications running within Hadoop. It functions independently and is decoupled from the resource management framework of Hadoop, i.e., the YARN infrastructure.

HDFS comprises a single **NameNode** and multiple **DataNodes** as shown in Figure 6.15. The NameNode stores the metadata, while the DataNodes store the data. A record called **inode** on the NameNode represents a file or directory and stores information such as permission, access time, etc.

A file within HDFS is broken down into several chunks or blocks and the chunks are distributed across the cluster nodes to be stored on the DataNodes. The blocks are also replicated and the copies are distributed in such a way that at least another node always maintains a copy of each block. This enables the system to find another location of the data, when a particular node storing the data crashes. Thus, processing of the data continues even though there is a failure of one or more nodes. The NameNode keeps track of the number of replicas of a block. When a replica of a block is lost due to node failure, the NameNode creates another replica of it. The *namespace* tree is maintained on the NameNode along with the mapping of blocks onto the DataNodes.

The specific features that ensure efficient storage and availability of data in the Hadoop cluster include:

- While scheduling tasks, HDFS takes into account the physical location of the node.

- Tasks or processes are moved to the data and the tasks are executed on the node where data (the block) resides. This reduces the number of packet movements through the network.

- The file system is monitored on a regular basis and data is rearranged on different nodes to maintain the balance.

- In the case of any error, the previous version of HDFS is rolled back after an upgrade.

- A **Standby NameNode** is configured to provide redundancy and availability.

6.6.4   MapReduce Framework

An application in Hadoop runs as a **job**. The master within the MapReduce framework is called the **MRAppMaster**. The execution of the job is carried out in two phases: i) the *map* phase, and ii) the *reduce* phase. However, these two phases may overlap.

At the beginning of a *map* phase, an application is submitted by the client that contains a configuration file, the *map()* implementation, the *reduce()* implementation, combiner implementation, the input directory on HDFS (or on some other file system), and the output directory where the resulting data will be stored. Each *map()* task is assigned with an input split or **map split** which contains a portion of the data. Size of the input split can be user-defined or can be of the default size as defined by the file system (e.g., HDFS block size is 64MB). The number of *map()* tasks depends on the number of files (and the number of blocks) or the number of map splits inside the input directory.

The MapReduce Application Master sends a request to the ResourceManager asking for a container. The Resource Scheduler contacts the NodeManagers to allocate the container either on the same node where the data is located, or on a node sharing the same rack as the node storing the data. However, the Resource Scheduler can also ignore the data locality and allocate the container on a different node by contacting its NodeManager. The *map()* task is initiated after allocation of the container.

Each *map()* task has the following phases:

1. during the INIT phase the task is set up;

2. during the EXECUTION phase, the *map()* function is executed for each (key, value) tuple inside the map split;

3. the output of the *map()* function is stored in an in-memory buffer and when this buffer becomes full, the data is removed from the buffer — this phase is called the SPILLING phase;

4. finally, in the SHUFFLE phase, all the *map()* outputs are sorted and merged based on the key and prepared for the reduce phase.

After the shuffle phase, each *reduce*() task will have a unique key and a list of values corresponding to that key. The number of *reduce*() tasks for the job is decided by the configuration parameter, which is usually input by the user.

6.6.5   Hadoop Common

Hadoop Common is central to the Hadoop software framework. It is a kernel that provides the essential utilities and libraries. Hadoop Common creates an abstraction of the underlying operating system and its file system. It also contains the necessary JAR (Java Archive) files and the scripts required to start Hadoop. Hadoop Common is also known as Hadoop Core.

6.6.6   Hadoop Performance

MapReduce on Hadoop offers two major advantages for its users:

1. Parallel processing of the splitted jobs across several computers on a Hadoop cluster.
2. Exploiting data locality by moving the computation close to the data.

However, there are many performance problems with the current implementation of Hadoop. Network traffic and I/O are the causes of major performance problems. Hadoop cannot process small-sized files efficiently. It can process only large-sized files. Even with large files, it often fails to offer the desired efficiency. Setting up the Hadoop system and maintaining it is a complex task because of the inherent complexity within the framework. It is implemented in Java and therefore is not scalable to the extent required for big data problems. The HDFS and MapReduce are not optimised for performance and therefore cannot perform well with different types of applications [12].

6.7   Hadoop Ecosystem

A number of tools, platforms, and frameworks are provided within the Hadoop ecosystem in order to handle the big data challenges [13]. In the previous section, we already discussed YARN, HDFS, and MapReduce. Some other useful components are given below:

- ZooKeeper and Ambari for managing cluster

- Oozie for job scheduling

- Solr and Lucene for searching and indexing

- Spark for in-memory data processing

- PIG, HIVE, and DRILL for data processing services using SQL-like query

- HBase as NoSQL database

- Mahout and Spark MLlib as a machine learning framework

Some of the above-mentioned components are discussed in detail in the following subsections. Some others, such as HBase, is discussed in Chapter 7

6.7.1   Apache Spark

On the homepage of Apache Spark, it is claimed that users may use Spark to "run programs up to 100 times faster than Hadoop MapReduce in memory, or 10 times faster on disk" [15] [8]. Spark reduces the number of read/write operations to disk and stores the intermediate data in the memory. Thus, it is claimed that Spark runs much faster compared to Hadoop MapReduce framework.

The other advantage of Spark is that it provides built-in APIs to support multiple languages, including Java, Scala, and Python. Further, in addition to the MapReduce programming paradigm, Spark also provides support for SQL queries and machine learning and graph algorithms.

Spark Deployment

There are three possible ways of deploying Spark on Hadoop. First of all, Spark can be deployed in standalone mode on top of HDFS, and Spark and MapReduce can both run simultaneously on a cluster. Spark can also be installed on top of YARN and thus can be integrated with the Hadoop stack. Spark can also be run within the MapReduce framework of Hadoop.

The following components are included in a Spark deployment:

1. Apache Spark Core — the execution engine with other required functionalities

2. Spark SQL — a component on top of Spark Core that provides support for accessing structured and semi-structured data.

3. Spark Streaming — a component to support analysis of streaming data.

4. MLlib — a distributed machine learning framework.

5. GraphX — a distributed graph-processing framework. It provides API for expressing graph computation to model the user-defined graphs.

Functioning of Spark

In every Spark application, the main function defined by the user runs as a driver program. The driver program executes parallel operations on a cluster. Functioning of Spark depends on the creation of a *Resilient Distributed Dataset* (RDD). RDD is a collection of elements that can be partitioned across a cluster and operated on in parallel. RDD can be created either by parallelising an existing collection in the driver program, or referencing a dataset in an external storage system.

Two types of operations on RDDs are supported: (i) transformations, which create a new dataset from an existing one, and (ii) actions, which compute a value from the dataset. An example of transformation is *map*, which creates a new RDD representing the results. On the other hand, *reduce* is an example of an action that aggregates all the elements of the RDD using a given function and returns the final result to the driver program. While, RDDs can contain any type of objects, Spark provides a few special operations to work on RDDs of key-value pairs. An example of such operations is grouping or aggregating the elements by a key.

Spark also allows the use of shared variables in parallel operations. A variable may be shared across tasks, or between tasks and the driver program. A shared variable can be (i) a broadcast variable, which is placed as a read-only variable in the cache memory of each machine, and (ii) an accumulator variable, which can be used in some associative and commutative operations to obtain a result.

6.7.2   Apache ZooKeeper

Apache ZooKeeper coordinates the Hadoop jobs and other required services within a Hadoop Ecosystem. ZooKeeper can maintain configuration information, and provide distributed synchronisation of data, along with grouping and naming of the services.

ZooKeeper coordinates distributed processes through a shared hierarchical name space of data registers. The registers, which are similar to file systems, are called **znodes**.

A name in ZooKeeper is a sequence of path elements separated by a slash ('/'). Every znode is identified by a path and is a child of a node whose path is a prefix of the znode with one element less. As in the case of a standard file system, the root ('/') has no parent. Also, a znode with children cannot be deleted.

Every znode has data associated with it. It stores coordination data, such as status information, configuration, location information, etc.

ZooKeeper service is replicated over a set of machines which together constitute the service. All these servers must know each other. Each server maintains an in-memory image of the data tree along with transaction log. A client must also have the list of servers, but it connects to only one server at a time through a TCP connection.

ZooKeeper provides its clients high throughput, low latency, highly available, and strictly ordered access to the znodes. Due to its improved performance, it can be used in large distributed systems. Because of its high availability, the problem due to a single point of failure can be avoided in big systems. Its strict ordering allows implementation of sophisticated synchronisation primitives at the client.

6.8 Streaming Data Processing

In the usual cases of healthcare scenarios, batch processing of data is more effective. Batch processing enables computation of or querying different sets of data. It usually involves computations using a large data set and enables deep analysis of big data sets. MapReduce-based systems are examples of platforms that support batch jobs. On the other hand, in many healthcare scenarios, such as in the case of continuous monitoring of patients, data is generated continuously from health sensors. Such continuous streams of data generated from many data sources (here sensors) are termed streaming data.

In contrast with batch processing, stream processing requires ingesting a sequence of data, and incrementally updating metrics, reports, and summary statistics in response to each arriving data record. The data is processed on a record-by-record basis or in small micro-batches. In some cases, data is also processed within a time window which slides through the data as new records are generated. Thus, while complex analysis is possible in the case of batch processing, streaming data processing only involves simple computation, like aggregation, filtering, etc.

The main challenges of streaming data processing is to maintain the ordering of the data as they are generated from various sources, to maintain data consistency, and to enable fast access to the data. The results of processing should also be stored back for future use. Deciding for how long the streaming records should be stored, i.e., their durability is also necessary. Scalability and fault tolerance are two other issues.

Several platforms have emerged that provide the necessary frameworks to build streaming data applications. These platforms include Apache Flume, Apache Storm, Apache Spark Streaming, Amazon Kinesis Streams, and Amazon Kinesis Firehose. Some of these platforms are discussed in this section.

6.8.1 Apache Flume

Apache Flume [16] [9] supports collection and aggregation of large amounts of streaming data from several distributed sources, and moving that data to a

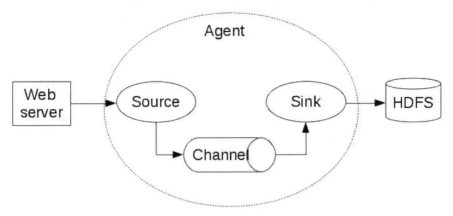

FIGURE 6.16: Apache Flume data model. [Source: https://flume.apache.org]

centralised data store. Typical sources of the streaming data are application logs, sensors, geo-location data, and social media. The different types of data can be sent to Hadoop for future analysis. Each data unit in Flume is treated as an *event*. An event carries an array of bytes as payload and an optional set of attributes as header. A process known as *Flume agent* helps to flow an event from an external source to an external destination. Three components within Flume perform the task of delivering the events: these are *source, channel,* and *sink*.

A source receives events from the external source, and stores the event into one or more channels. A channel is like a temporary buffer which stores the event until it is consumed by a sink. The sink removes the event from the channel and sends it to an external repository. An example of channel is *FileChannel*, which uses a local filesystem for storage. The event may also be forwarded to the source at the next hop of the flow. The dataflow model within Flume is shown in Figure 6.16.

Apache claims Flume is reliable because it uses a transactional approach to guarantee the reliable delivery of events [16]. Events are delivered by a sink either to the source within the agent at the next hop or to the final repository. The delivery happens in the form of a transaction, and when two agents are involved in the process, the sink from the previous hop and the source of the next hop keep their transactions open to ensure that the event data is safely stored in the channel of the next hop. A sink removes the event from its channel only when it is stored in the channel of the next agent. Such point-to-point flow ensures end-to-end reliability of the flow. Flume is scalable horizontally to ingest new data streams and additional volumes as needed. In other words, in order to improve the performance of Flume, the number of machines on which Flume is deployed needs to be increased. The components within the Flume agent work asynchronously and therefore, the platform can

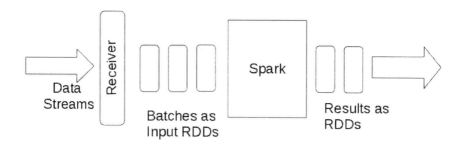

FIGURE 6.17: Apache Spark Streaming

handle transient spikes, i.e., when the rate of incoming data exceeds the rate at which data can be written to the destination.

6.8.2 Spark Streaming

Spark Streaming provides a set of APIs for stream processing that allows the users to write streaming jobs in the same way as they write the batch jobs. Spark Streaming receives data streams from input sources, processes them on a cluster, and then sends the results to databases or to dashboards. It can read data from HDFS, Flume, Kafka, Twitter, etc. One can also define his or her own custom data sources.

Spark Streaming also allows to join streams against historical data and run ad-hoc queries on stream state. Interactive applications can be developed along with analytic jobs. Languages which can be used for Spark Streaming are Java, Scala, and Python. While running on Spark, it is possible to reuse the same code for batch processing as in Spark Streaming.

In Spark Streaming, first the data streams are divided into batches of RDDs, each with a duration of only few seconds. The batches are processed using RDD operations and the results are also forwarded as batches of RDDs, as shown in Figure 6.17.

The programming model of Spark Streaming is based on a high-level abstraction known as *discretized stream* or *DStream*. It represents a continuous stream of data which is basically a sequence of RDDs.

Spark Streaming can be deployed on top of the standalone cluster mode of Spark. A local run mode is supported for development. Spark Streaming uses ZooKeeper and HDFS for resource management and storage of data with high availability.

6.8.3   Amazon Kinesis Streaming Data Platform

Amazon Kinesis Steaming Data Platform is built with several components, such as *Amazon Kinesis Streams*, *Amazon Kinesis Data Firehose*, and *Amazon Kinesis Data Analytics*.

Amazon Kinesis Streams allows a user to develop applications for collecting, processing, and analysing high throughput streaming data. Real-time data, such as video, audio, application logs, website clickstreams, and data produced by sensors and IoT devices can be consumed by Amazon Kinesis applications and can be used for machine learning, analytics, and other applications. A user application is able to process the data as soon as it arrives without keeping the user waiting till the end of the data stream, thereby enabling the user to respond instantly.

Amazon Kinesis Data Firehose, another component of the Amazon streaming data platform, provides support for delivering real-time streaming data to destination, such as Amazon Simple Storage Service or Amazon S3, etc. The user just needs to configure the data producers to send data to Kinesis Data Firehose. Firehose then automatically sends the data to the destination as specified by the user. Kinesis Data Firehose can also perform certain transformations on the user data before delivering it. For example, it can compress or encrypt data before delivering it to the destination.

Additionally, *Amazon Kinesis Data Analytics* is used for processing data streams in real time using simple query languages, such as SQL.

6.9   Chapter Notes

This chapter provides an overview of the high performance architectures and computational models for processing big data. It begins with the discussion of various performance issues which are considered for high performance computing. The chapter then introduces different parallel architectural models including recent developments, such as Cluster Computing and GPU Computing. The chapter also holds a discussion on parallel programming models which are frequently used for programming parallel computers. An overview of *MapReduce* programming is given in this chapter, because of its recent popularity in big data processing.

The chapter also briefly describes the tools for processing big data. Hadoop, being the most popular platform in this family, provides several tools in this regard. Hadoop is based on a MapReduce framework.

Hadoop is mainly meant for batch data processing. On the other hand, in helthcare scenarios, streaming data processing is another important requirement. A preliminary discussion on the processing of streaming data is introduced in this chapter and some popular tools for processing of streaming data are discussed.

References

[1] G. Amdahl. Validity of the single-processor approach to achieving large-scale computing capabilities. In *AFIPS '67 (Spring) Proceedings of the spring joint computer conference*, volume 38, pages 483–485, April 1967.

[2] N. Balakrishnan, T. Bytheway, L. Carata, O. R. A. Chick, J. Snee, S. Akoush, R. Sohan, M. Seltzer, and A. Hopper. Recent advances in computer architecture: the opportunities and challenges for provenance. In *Proceedings of the 7th USENIX Conference on Theory and Practice of Provenance (TaPP'15)*. USENIX Association, Berkeley, CA, USA, 2015.

[3] R. Balasubramonian, J. Chang, T. Manning, J. H. Moreno, R. Murphy, R. Nair, and S. Swanson. Near-Data Processing: Insights from a MICRO-46 Workshop. *IEEE Micro*, 34(4):36–42, July–August 2014.

[4] L. A. Barroso, J. Dean, and U. Holzle. Web search for a planet: The Google cluster architecture. *IEEE Micro*, 23(2):22–28, March 2003.

[5] E. Coppa. Hadoop Internals. Website: http://ercoppa.github.io/HadoopInternals/, 2017.

[6] J. Dean and S. Ghemawat. MapReduce: Simplified Data Processing on Large Clusters. In *Proceedings of the 6th Conference on Symposium on Opearting Systems Design & Implementation - Volume 6*, OSDI'04, pages 10–10, Berkeley, CA, USA, 2004. USENIX Association.

[7] J. Dean and S. Ghemawat. MapReduce: Simplified Data Processing on Large Clusters. *Communications of the ACM*, 51(1):107–113, 2008.

[8] S. Farook, G. Lakshmi Narayana, and B. Tarakeswara Rao. Spark is superior to Map Reduce over Big Data. *International Journal of Computer Applications*, 133(1):13–16, January 2016. Published by Foundation of Computer Science (FCS), NY, USA.

[9] Hortonworks. Apache Flume. Website: https://hortonworks.com/apache/flume/.

[10] NVIDIA. *NVIDIA CUDA Compute Unified Device Architecture Programming Guide*, 1.0 edition.

[11] G. F. Pfister. *In Search of Clusters*. Prentice Hall Inc., 2nd edition, 1998.

[12] H. S. Ray, K. Naguri, P. Sil Sen, and N. Mukherjee. Comparative Study of Query Performance in a Remote Health Framework using Cassandra and Hadoop. In *Proceedings of the 9th International Joint Conference on Biomedical Engineering Systems and Technologies (BIOSTEC 2016)– Volume 5: HEALTHINF, Rome, Italy, February 21–23, 2016*, pages 330–337, 2016.

[13] S. Sinha. Hadoop Ecosystem: Hadoop Tools for Crunching Big Data. Website: `https://www.edureka.co/blog/hadoop-ecosystem`, 2016.

[14] A. Snell. Beyond Beowulf: Clusters, Cores, and a New Era of TOP500, Intersect360 Research. Website: `https://www.top500.org/news/beyond-beowulf-clusters-cores-and-a-new-era-of-top500/`, November 2014.

[15] Hadoop Team. Spark vs. Hadoop – Who Wins? Website: `hadoopinrealworld.com/spark-vs-hadoop-who-wins`.

[16] The Apache Flume Team. Apache Flume. Website: `https://flume.apache.org/`.

[17] B. Wilkinson and M. Allen. *Parallel Programming: Techniques and Applications using Networked Workstations and Parallel Computers*. Pearson, 2nd edition, 2007.

[18] J. Zhao and J. Pjesivac-Grbovic. MapReduce: The programming model and practice. Website: `https://research.google.com/archive/papers/mapreduce-sigmetrics09-tutorial.pdf`, 2009. SIGMETRICS'09 Tutorial.

7

Big Data Storage

CONTENTS

7.1	Introduction	....	163
7.2	Structured vs. Unstructured Data	....	164
7.3	Problems with Relational Databases	....	165
7.4	NoSQL Databases	....	166
7.5	Document-oriented Databases	....	168
	7.5.1	MongoDB	169
	7.5.2	Apache CouchDB	173
7.6	Column-oriented Databases	....	174
	7.6.1	Apache Cassandra	174
	7.6.2	Apache HBase	179
7.7	Graph Databases	....	181
	7.7.1	Neo4j	181
7.8	Health Data Storage: A Case Study	....	184
7.9	Chapter Notes	....	188

7.1 Introduction

Some recent studies reveal interesting facts [14] and statistics about big data. Some of the facts are: '2.7 Zetabytes of data exist in the digital universe today', 'Facebook stores, accesses, and analyses 30+ Petabytes of user generated data', 'Walmart handles more than 1 million customer transactions every hour, which is imported into databases estimated to contain more than 2.5 petabytes of data', 'more than 5 billion people are calling, texting, tweeting and browsing on mobile phones worldwide' and so on. Storing and managing such voluminous data is one of the most important challenges in today's computer science research. There is no doubt that this vast amount of data is unstructured or semi-structured. Since the mid-1970s, when databases came into play, business intelligence mostly relied on structured databases (more specifically, relational databases). However, the huge amount data that is being generated every day in contemporary times from several data sources is primarily unstructured. People write emails, generate corporate documents, and create news, blog articles and web pages. Every day, social networks generate vast amounts of data. Sensors, when deployed for continuous monitoring or event-based monitoring for various applications, generate data, which is also mostly unstructured.

7.2   Structured vs. Unstructured Data

Seth Grimes, an industry analyst on the confluence of structured and unstructured data sources, once stated in an article [10]: "80% of business-relevant information originates in unstructured form, primarily text". Anant Jhingran of IBM Research claims that amount of unstructured data is no less than 85%. Contradicting these claims, Philip Russom of the Data Warehousing Institute says: "structured data in first place at 47%, trailed by unstructured (31%) and semi-structured data (22%)". His statement is based on an unstructured-data study in 2006. In other words, unstructured and semi-structured data beat structured data in volume amounting to 53% of the data that the world generates. Whatever the exact percentage of unstructured data which is being generated and used for business intelligence and other purposes, there is no doubt that the amount of unstructured data is much more compared to structured data.

There is also a debate regarding the term 'unstructured'. Some technologists claim that although in some cases structure may not be clearly identified, it can still be implicitly defined, and therefore, it should not be labeled unstructured. As one such example, they cite the case of 'email'. However, a more acceptable definition of 'unstructured' is as follows: if data has some form of structure but is not helpful to the processing task at hand, it may still be characterised as 'unstructured' [17]. Thus, although email messages may have some implied structure, presently available data mining tools cannot parse the emails to extract useful information. Therefore, emails are also treated as unstructured data. Not just emails, but word processing files, PDF files, spreadsheets, digital images, videos, audios, and social media posts are treated as unstructured data. Some more facts related to unstructured data are as follows: 'YouTube users upload 48 hours of new video every minute of the day', '571 new websites are created every minute of the day', 'different brands and organizations on Facebook receive 34,722 "Likes" every minute of the day', '100 terabytes of data uploaded daily to Facebook' and according to Twitters own research in early 2012, 'roughly 175 million tweets are made every day'.

Chapter 3 already explained why health data is big data. Health data is also unstructured data. Most EHRs now contain quantitative data (e.g., laboratory results as numeric or literal values), qualitative data (e.g., text-based documents and demographics), and transactional data (e.g., a record of medication delivery). However, much of this data is currently perceived as a by-product of healthcare delivery. There are other sources of information which are nowadays essential for improving the efficiency in healthcare delivery. The data sources include text documents, clinical reports, images, videos, and audios. This data is unstructured and the amount of such data generated every day is huge.

7.3 Problems with Relational Databases

Storing large amounts of big data in relational databases is not efficient for the following reasons [8]:

- Relational databases require predefined schemas before loading data. When a new data source is added in the system, it becomes difficult to change the schema.

- In the modern applications, changes in the data model are very common. This is because the requirements may change rapidly, and accordingly, the changes need to be reflected in the data model. However, while using relational databases, even a small change like adding or replacing a column in a table might be expensive and time consuming.

- The table structure of a relational database with rows and columns is designed for storing sets of values. On the other hand, unstructured data is not only values, but contains much more information than that. For example, it may contain relationships (of a patient to family members or care providers, to symptoms and medications), geospatial data (addresses), metadata (provenance, security attributes), images (CT scan reports), and free text (doctors' notes, transcripts).

  - Relational databases are not designed for handling heterogeneous formats of data.

  - Relational databases become inefficient and ineffective to store time-varying data.

- Relational databases cannot handle mixed workloads. For example, for transactional workloads and for analytical workloads, relational database architectures must be designed differently.

- Modern applications use object-oriented programming languages. Data structures are treated as 'objects' encapsulating both data and methods. However, relational databases are not equipped to handle data in this manner and are therefore not efficient for modern applications.

- Achieving scalability and elasticity is a big challenge for relational databases.

– Relational databases are designed to run on a single server in order to maintain the integrity of the table mappings and avoid the problems of distributed computing. Therefore, if the system needs to scale up, new hardware with higher power needs to be procured at much higher cost.

– Scaling down is practically impossible for relational databases.

An example of healthcare data may be considered to explain the problem with the rigid, schema-based approach of relational databases. The advice of a doctor to a patient can include one or more of the following items: (i) medication for a specified period of time, (ii) pathological tests, (iii) diagnostic tests like MRI, CT-Scan, etc., (iv) advice related to lifestyle, nutrition etc., (v) referral to a specialist doctor (establishing a new relationship), and so on. Such advice is itself too complex to be stored in a relational database. If the patient returns to the same doctor with test reports and also with further description about his or her health, the reports and the state of his or her health are also to be stored in the database for future reference. The reports may contain numeric or text data, images, graphs, and many other data in a variety of formats. Handling such complicated data models is not possible using relational databases.

Even if only the diagnostics test reports of the patients are stored in a table in relational databases, considering the heterogeneity of such reports, the table becomes too complex for efficient handling. The following few options are considered in such cases:

1. A very wide table with hundreds of fields may be created for any possible attributes related to the medical tests, but for most tests most of these fields will be NULL.

2. A separate table for each product test category may be created.

3. A huge table with the columns test name, test attribute, and value may be created, mapping all the attributes to the values. But again, the heterogeneous structure of the data will be difficult to store with this mapping.

All three options mentioned above are valid, but none of them is really satisfying in terms of effectiveness and flexibility.

Thus, more flexible data models and data storage systems, which can overcome the above-mentioned impedance, and work as better matches for modern application development, are required.

7.4 NoSQL Databases

The term 'NoSQL' was used by Carlo Strozzi when he first introduced a lightweight open source relational database, namely 'NoSQL' [18]. Later, the term has become popular to describe the family of databases which are 'Non-SQL' or 'Not Only SQL' and non-relational. This family of databases provide storage and retrieval mechanisms, with less constrained consistency models than traditional relational databases [11].

Unlike relational databases, NoSQL databases do not store data in tables. Instead, they are either document-oriented or store data in some other flexible and scalable formats. Some of the key differences between relational databases and NoSQL databases are given in Table 7.1.

TABLE 7.1: Key differences between relational and NoSQL databases

Relational Database	NoSQL Database
Supports powerful query language	Supports simple query language
It has a fixed schema	No fixed schema
Follows ACID Property (Atomicity, Consistency, Isolation, and Durability)	It is only 'eventually consistent'
Supports transactions	Does not support transactions

NoSQL databases exist in the following categories:

- *Key-value stores*

  Key-value databases store key-value pairs, i.e., each unique key is associated with the values. For the inherent simplicity of the model, it can be highly scalable and perform much better than many other models for certain applications. Example of these databases include **Azure** and **Riak**.

- *Document databases*

  Document databases store semi-structured data and descriptions of that data in document format. Unstructured data can be stored in a single document that can be easily found. However, the data is not necessarily categorized into fields like relational databases. Such types of storage systems store data in bulk and therefore require additional processing effort and more storage compared to simple relational databases. Computing platforms like Hadoop may be used in conjunction with NoSQL databases for processing the data.

  Use of document databases has increased in the development of modern web applications and mobile applications which are written in JavaScript using data interchange formats like JSON (JavaScript Object Notation) [1] or XML

---

[1]JavaScript Object Notation or JSON is a human-readable, plain text format for expressing structured data.

and other data formats. JSON is currently supported in many programming languages. **CouchDB**, **DocumentDB**, **MarkLogic**, and **MongoDB** are examples of document databases.

- *Wide-column stores*

  In such types of databases, data tables are organised as columns instead of rows. When data is stored in wide-column stores, queries to large data volumes can be made faster than conventional relational databases. Some wide-column databases support SQL queries as well. **Cassandra**, **Google BigTable**, and **HBase** are examples of wide-column stores.

- *Graph stores*

  Data is organized as nodes. A node actually stores the data which can be represented in a single record in a relational database. The edges connecting these nodes represent the relationships between these records. Using the edges, a graph database can support richer representations of data relationships. Because of its structure, the graph data model can evolve over time and use. Examples of graph databases include **AllegroGraph**, **IBM Graph**, **Neo4j**, and **Titan**.

- *Data structure stores*

  Data structure stores are conceptually similar to key-value stores. However, while in traditional key-value stores, keys in string format are associated with string values, in data structure stores the value is not limited to a simple string, but can also hold more complex data structures. **Redis** is an example of such type of storage.

  In the following sections, some of the popular NoSQL databases are described.

7.5   Document-oriented Databases

Unlike relational databases, document-oriented databases are not structured in the form of tables containing rows. Rather, documents are used as storage structures in these databases. The documents are used for storing, retrieving and managing semi-structured data. Thus, the databases have flexible schema and data models in contrast with the fixed schema in relational databases.

Usually, XML, JSON, and BSON [2] documents are used for storing data.

---

[2]BSON or Binary JSON is a binary-encoded serialisation of JSON-like documents.

Nevertheless, PDFs or other kinds of documents may also be stored. As the databases support flexible schema, the documents can have similar or different structures. Each document contains a description of the data type and a value for that description. Whenever a new data type is required to be added to the database, there is no need to change the entire structure; rather this modification can be done just by adding an object to the database. Documents are grouped into *collections*. Queries can be issued to search the collections of documents for retrieving certain data. In this section, two document-oriented databases are discussed.

7.5.1   MongoDB

MongoDB is one of the popular documented-oriented databases. The MongoDB database is organized as follows.

A single MongoDB server stores multiple databases. The largest container in the MongoDB database is a *collection*. A MongoDB database is developed as a collection of documents. Although a collection resembles a relational database table, it does not enforce a fixed schema. The documents in a collection can have different fields.

MongoDB Data Model

The basic unit in the database is a *document*, which is analogous to the rows in relational databases. However, unlike the rows or tuples in relational databases, a document has a dynamic schema, i.e., fields may be added on the fly. The fields in the documents in a collection may vary and even the common fields in a collection of documents can store different types of data. A document in MongoDB is stored as a set of key-value pairs. An _id field is added by MongoDB to uniquely identify the document in the collection. The _id field is the primary key in a document. If the user defines a document without an _id field, MongoDB automatically adds the field.

The MongoDB data model enables the user to store arrays, and other more complex structures; it also extends support for hierarchical relationships.

Relationships between Data

The relationships between documents in MongoDB databases can be established in two ways: using *references* or using *embedded documents*.

- *References* — References resemble foreign keys in relational databases. Figure 7.1 depicts one such relationship. Here the 'Patient' document contains a few details of the patient, including name, name of the care-person at home, address, contact number, etc. The 'DemographicInfo' document includes age, sex, education level, income level, marital status, occupation, religion, etc. The 'BasicClinicalParameters' document includes basic clinical parameters, such as blood group, height, weight, etc. The segregation of demographic information from clinical parameters helps to preserve privacy in the data model.

Two types of references are supported:

1. A 'manual reference' stores the *_id* field of one document in another document as a reference.

2. A 'DBRef' relates one document to another using the value of its *_id* field, collection name, and its database name (optional). Thus, using DBRefs, documents owned by multiple collections can be linked with documents from a single collection.

However, manual references can be used in most cases and there is little requirement of using DBRefs.

- *Embedded Documents* — Embedded documents impose a hierarchical structure while storing related data in multiple related sub-documents stored within a single document. Document structure can be embedded in a field or array within a document. Figure 7.2 shows an embedded document structure for 'patient', 'DemographicInfo', and BasicClinicalParameters.

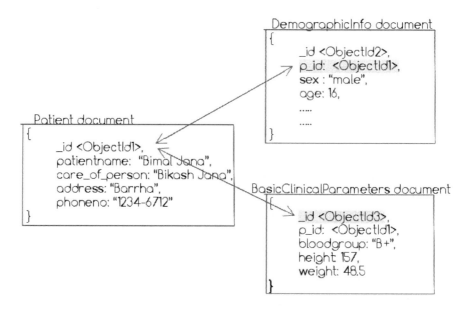

FIGURE 7.1: MongoDB referencing relationship between data

Write Operations in MongoDB

'Write' operations in MongoDB are atomic, which means that a single 'write' operation affects only one document in a collection. If modification of more

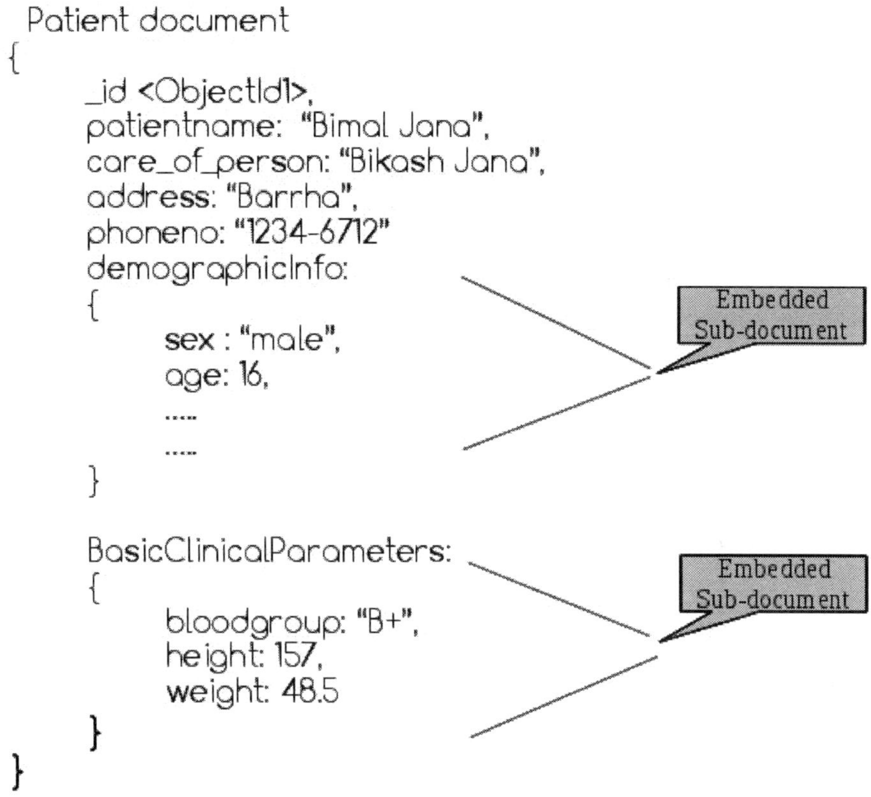

```
Patient document
{
      _id <ObjectId1>,
      patientname: "Bimal Jana",
      care_of_person: "Bikash Jana",
      address: "Barrha",
      phoneno: "1234-6712"
      demographicInfo:
      {
            sex : "male",
            age: 16,

            .....

            .....
      }

BasicClinicalParameters:
{
      bloodgroup: "B+",
      height: 157,
      weight: 48.5
}
}
```

Embedded Sub-document

Embedded Sub-document

FIGURE 7.2: MongoDB embedded documents

than a single document in a collection is necessary, operation takes place on one document at a time. Thus, for queries with *references*, additional queries are needed to return the results from multiple related documents.

However, when all related data are embedded in a single document, a single 'write' operation can be used to update or insert all data related to an entity. Thus, when atomic updates are necessary, it must be ensured that all fields with atomic dependency requirements should be stored in the same document.

Scalability, Availability, and Performance

In order to handle very large databases, a collection can be partitioned and distributed for storage across a number of *mongod* instances or shards on multiple nodes within a cluster. A *shard key* is used for partitioning the collection. A sharded collection has only one shard key. The choice of shard key is important as it affects the performance, efficiency, and horizontal scalability of the database. Once a shard key is chosen, it cannot be changed.

Availability of data is achieved by creating a *replica set*. A *replica set* is a group of *mongod* instances that maintain the same data set. It contains several nodes storing data, and optionally, a node for arbitration. Among the data nodes, one node is designated as the primary node and others as secondary nodes. All 'write' operations are sent to the primary node. All changes in the data are recorded in an operation log known as the *oplog*. The secondary nodes replicate the oplog and apply the changes to the data in order to maintain consistency among the replications. When the primary node is not available, an eligible secondary node is elected through an election procedure as the new primary node. Arbiters are not used to store data, rather they are used to maintain a quorum in a replica set by responding to heartbeat and election requests by other replica set members.

All reads are made from the primary node. However, the users can specify a preferred node from the replica set to send read operations.

Indexes are used to improve performance for common queries. Indexes are built on fields which frequently appear in queries. For all documents, a unique index is automatically created on the _id field.

Interfacing with MongoDB

An interactive JavaScript interface to MongoDB for querying and updating data is provided by the mongo shell. It is also used for administrative operations.

The query language for MongoDB has much difference with SQL. It has its own syntax which is similar to dot notation for JavaScript arrays. Other scripting languages like python, PHP, or perl are also supported; however, the respective language interpreters need to be installed in each case.

Data Aggregation

MongoDB supports three types of *aggregation* operations:

- the aggregation pipeline — here documents are input to a multi-stage pipeline which transforms the input into an aggregated result, e.g., grouping and sorting of documents.

- the map-reduce function — similar to other map-reduce tools. Here map-reduce operations implement a map phase to process each document and emit one or more objects for each input document, and a reduce phase to combine the output of the map operation.

- single purpose aggregation methods — these operations aggregate documents from a single collection, e.g., return the 'count' of documents, or return the number of distinct documents, etc.

Further Reading

Further details of data storage and usage of MongoDB databases may be found in [4] [5] [23].

7.5.2 Apache CouchDB

CouchDB is another document-oriented database. Initially developed by Damien Katz in 2005, it became an Apache project in 2008. CouchDB primarily stores JSON documents.

CouchDB Data Model

The primary unit for data storage in the CouchDB database is a document. Documents consist of fields and attachments. Like other semi-structured NoSQL databases, CouchDB also does not have any fixed schema. Therefore, there can be any number of fields in the document. Fields have unique names and are associated with values of varying types (text, number, boolean, lists, etc.). The size of the text or number of elements in the list can be unlimited.

Documents also contain metadata and the metadata revision information. The metadata is simply a set of attributes describing the document. The attribute names begin with an '_', such as '_id', '_rev', and '_attachments'.

Indexing: A B-tree index is created for the documents with *DocID* and a *sequenceID*. Each update to a database instance generates a new sequenceID, which is used to determine the incremental changes in the database. The indexes are updated simultaneously when documents are saved or deleted.

Views: CouchDB allows users to dynamically create *views* on top of the document database. Users can use these *views* to aggregate or join the database documents or generate reports on the documents. As the view definitions are virtual and they are created dynamically, no changes are made on the actual physical documents.

ACID Properties

The four properties, namely 'Atomicity', 'Consistency', 'Isolation' and 'Durability', also known as ACID properties, are implemented in CouchDB. Document updates follow *atomicity*, i.e., either the changes are saved completely or not saved at all. At no point of time will the database have any partially saved or edited documents. Updates in the documents, i.e., 'add', 'edit' and 'delete' are serialised. However, 'read' operations may be concurrently issued. A Multi-Version Concurrency Control (MVCC) technique[3] is used to support any number of clients reading documents without waiting or being interrupted by concurrent 'write' operations.

When documents are committed to disk, the metadata and fields are packed in buffers and sequentially stored onto the disk one after another. All data and associated indexes are flushed onto disk, and finally, each such commit operation leaves the database in a consistent state.

---

[3]MVCC maintains multiple copies of each data item. Thus, each user sees a snapshot of the database at a particular instant of time. Any changes made by a 'write' operation will not be seen by other users until it is committed.

Data Replication

The replication mechanism allows CouchDB to maintain two (or more) copies of the same database, either on the same server or on different servers. Any change in one database is later reflected in the other copy using a bi-directional replication mechanism. The replication process is incremental, i.e., only the updates since the last replication are considered and sent to the other database, in a bi-directional manner. The sequenceID, mentioned earlier, is used for incremental replication. The replication mechanism allows the users to update the copies of the databases offline and synchronise the copies to obtain updated replicas of the databases.

Interfacing with CouchDB

CouchDB provides RESTful HTTP APIs for any addition, updating, and deletion operations in the database documents.

Further Reading

CouchDB resources and tutorials may be found in [2] [21]. Readers may also refer to Couchbase, another JSON-based document store derived from CouchDB with a Memcached-compatible interface[4].

7.6 Column-oriented Databases

In the column-oriented databases , data is stored in columns, not in rows. A column is stored in sequential blocks, either on disk or in-memory. For analytical queries, such as aggregate operations involving a small number of columns, these databases outperform other row-oriented databases. Insertion, updating or retrieval of a single record is slow in these databases. Nevertheless, in the case of the applications that mostly deal with time series data, these data stores perform very well, as new data is only appended to the end of the table. In this section, two column-oriented databases are described.

7.6.1 Apache Cassandra

Apache Cassandra [1] is an open source, distributed, and decentralised storage system. Cassandra accommodates structured, semi-structured, and unstructured data formats. It can also dynamically accommodate changes in the data structures according to the user's need. Cassandra provides a flexible way of distributing data by replicating data across multiple computational nodes.

---

[4]Memcached refers to an in-memory key-value store for small chunks of data which are obtained from the results of database calls, API calls, or page rendering.

Cassandra is deployed as a peer-to-peer distributed system across several nodes. Data is distributed among the cluster of nodes. Each node in a cluster, despite being interconnected with other nodes, plays the same independent role of a peer. Each node in a cluster can accept 'read' and 'write' requests, regardless of where the data is actually located in the cluster. When a node goes down, 'read' or 'write' requests can be served from other nodes in the network.

When Cassandra is deployed in a data center environment, data must be replicated among the nodes to avoid any single point of failure. Cassandra may also be configured to work in a multi-data center environment. The distribution of data and replication of data are easily configurable.

Cassandra Data Model

The outermost container for data in Cassandra is *keyspace*. The concept of *keyspace* is similar to the *database* in relational model.

A *keyspace* contains one or more *column families*. A *column family* is a container of an ordered collection of rows. Each row is again an ordered collection of columns. A row is identified by a unique key (a string without a size limit), called *partition key* or *row key*. *Column families* may be compared with tables in relational model (Figure 7.3). Unlike relational databases, there is no fixed schema. Although column families are defined, the columns are not. A user can add any column to any column family at any time. Also, individual rows may not have all the columns. A column in Cassandra is a data structure with a *column name* (or key), a *value*, and a *time stamp* (Figure 7.4 (a)). Thus, instead of storing just rows and columns as in the two-dimensional tables in relational databases, Cassandra stores list of nested key-value pairs, i.e., in each row, there is a map of column keys and the corresponding values. Thus, it can avoid the requirement of a fixed schema. Further, the number of column keys is unbounded, thus enabling the user to use wide rows. A key can itself hold a value and the column can be valueless.

Cassandra also provides a special data structure, namely *superColumn*, which is also a key-value pair, but stores a map of sub-columns instead of a single column (Figure 7.4 (b)). One can create many sub-columns within a superColumn and have different numbers of them in different superColumns. A single query can fetch data from some or all sub-columns. However, use of superColumns is not encouraged in Cassandra. This is because use of superColumns often leads to inefficiencies. One reason behind this inefficiency is that the superColumns are implemented as a single column with the sub-columns serialised within it. Hence, in order to read one sub-column, Cassandra needs to deserialise the whole superColumn, which may be very inefficient in the case of large superColumns. The concept of *composite columns* may be used to replace superColumns.

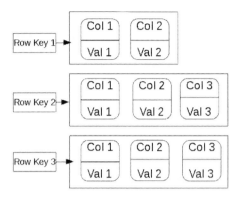

FIGURE 7.3: Cassandra column family [Source: [20]]

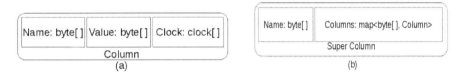

FIGURE 7.4: (a) Structure of a column, (b) Structure of a super column [Source: [20]]

Data Replication

Cassandra is designed for higher availability and partition tolerance (i.e., it falls in the 'AP' intersection of the CAP theorem, which states that any networked shared-data system can only guarantee two of the desired capabilities at the same time. These are 'C'onsistency, 'A'vailability and 'P'artition tolerance). Data partitioning and replication take place in the following manner.

As mentioned earlier, instances of Cassandra are installed on different nodes, forming a cluster. Data is distributed among the nodes using a consistent hashing algorithm and therefore the cluster is visualised as a ring. Each node in the ring stores a copy of the column families defined by the partition key. The partition keys are used by a hash function to decide the location of data and its replicas.

Each *keyspace* is associated with a parameter, called *the replication factor*, which is the number of machines in the cluster storing copies of the same data. For example, replication factor 1 means only one copy of each row will be stored, whereas if the factor is 2, each row will be stored on two nodes in the cluster. All replicas have the same importance. Cassandra allows users to configure the replication factor and the strategy.

The *replica placement strategy* is also defined for placing replicas in the ring. The strategy decides the distribution of the replicas across the nodes in the cluster depending on its topology. Currently, there are three strategies supported:

1. **Simple strategy** (earlier this was known as rack-unaware Strategy) — This strategy places replicas in a single data centre in a manner that is not aware of their placement on a data centre rack. This is the default strategy and may not always perform well, as the next node holding the replica can be on a different rack.

2. **Old network topology strategy** (formerly known as rack-aware strategy) — This strategy is used to distribute data across different racks in the same data centre. It is actually aware of the placement in data center racks.

3. **Network topology strategy** — This strategy helps the user to decide how replicas will be placed across the data centres. The user needs to supply parameters to indicate the desired replication strategy for each data centre.

Maintaining Consistency

With the updation of data, consistency among the replicas must also be maintained. Cassandra follows an *eventual consistency* model. A user can choose different consistency levels from low to high. Three levels of consistency are supported — ONE, QUORUM, and ALL. In the case of ALL, one 'write' operation will wait for the data to be written and confirmed by all nodes where the data has been replicated before replying to the client. QUORUM consistency means the majority of the nodes $(N/2+1)$ should write the data and confirm. Table 7.2 shows the 'Read' and 'Write' operations at the three consistency levels.

TABLE 7.2: Levels of Consistency

Level	Read	Write
ONE	Return data from nearest replica	Return when one replica commits data
QUORUM	Return most recent data from majority of replicas	Return when majority of replicas commit data
ALL	Return most recent data from all replicas	Return when all replicas commit data

Read and Write in Cassandra

Since there is no master node in Cassandra, a client can connect with any node in a cluster. The node that a client connects to is designated as the *coordinator* and it then becomes responsible for satisfying the client's request.

If the coordinator node itself does not hold the data on which a 'read' or 'write' operation is to be performed, it forwards the request to the nodes holding the data using messaging service in an asynchronous manner. The nodes are determined based on the partition key and the replication strategy. Depending on the levels of consistency, the coordinator decides how many nodes are to be communicated and how many nodes it needs to hear from before replying to the client.

Each node processes the request. If it is a 'write' request, every node which receives the request first writes the data in the *commit log*. After writing to the commit log, the data is written to a memory-resident data structure, known as the *mem-table*. As the mem-table is an in-memory structure, the writing to the commit log ensures durability of the 'write'. Therefore, the commit log provides support for crash recovery in case of node failure or other reasons for data losses from the mem-table. Data is only written to disk when the mem-table is flushed to disk. *SSTable* is a disk file to which the data is flushed from the mem-table when the contents of the mem-table reach a threshold value.

If it is a 'read' request, the coordinator determines the first replica and all other applicable replicas on the basis of the partition key and the replication strategy and replication factor. If the nodes, which are contacted by the co-ordinator, hold different versions of the replica, the coordinator returns the latest version to the client and issues a 'read repair' command to the node(s) having older copies of the replica. The command copies the newer version of the data to nodes with the older versions.

In order to reduce the number of disk accesses and to make any data access faster, Cassandra uses some cache-based mechanisms and in-memory indexes. *Bloom filter*, which is an in-memory structure (a special kind of cache) is one such mechanism. It provides non-deterministic algorithms for checking whether an element is a member of a set. Thus, it can check whether a row data exists in the mem-table before accessing the SSTables on disk. Bloom filters are accessed after every query. Cassandra also uses a type of index, known as *partition index*, that stores a list of partition keys and the start positions of the rows in the data file written on disk.

Gossip Protocol

Nodes in a cluster communicate using a peer-to-peer protocol known as *Gossip Protocol*. Based on this protocol, the nodes broadcast information about data and health of the nodes. However, each node does not need to talk with every other node to know something about them. Whenever a node communicates with another node, it not only provides information about its own status, it also provides the latest information about all nodes that it has communicated with recently. This process reduces the message exchange and increases the efficiency of information gathering.

Users can access Cassandra through its nodes using Cassandra Query Language (CQL). CQL treats the *keyspace* as a container of tables.

Further Reading

More resources and information on Cassandra can be found in [1] [20] [3] [13].

7.6.2 Apache HBase

HBase is another column-oriented database built on top of Hadoop. It has been designed to overcome many deficiencies of the *Hadoop Distributed File System* (HDFS).

HBase Data model

The HBase data model is similar to *Bigtable* offered by Google [9]. The data model in HBase consists of *tables* which are collections of rows. A *row* is identified by a rowkey. Data in a row are grouped together as *column families*. A *column family* contains one or more *columns* which are stored together. The logical view of a table is shown in Figure 7.5, with an example.

Row key	personal data				basic clinical parameters		
patient_id	name	village	age	sex	bloodgroup	height	weight
1	Bimal Jana	Barrha	16	male	B+	161	48
2	Gouri Sen	Bali	62	female	A+	159	54
3	Anita Ray	Suri	43	female	A+	160	62
4	Saral Bose	Bali	51	male	O	163	67

FIGURE 7.5: HBase table

A column is identified by a *column qualifier* consisting of the column family name concatenated with a colon followed by the column name. A *cell* stores data and is uniquely identified using rowkey, column family, and column qualifier. HBase maintains the versions of the data stored in a cell using timestamps. Thus, a combination of row, column, and version exactly specifies a cell. It is possible to create an unbounded number of cells with the same row and column, but with different versions. The cell address differs only in its version dimension. At the time of table creation, HBase allows users to specify the maximum (and minimum) number of versions to store for a given column.

In HBase, data is distributed among the nodes by splitting the tables. Tables are split into *regions* and regions are placed on the region servers. Regions are vertically divided by column families into *stores* and are saved as files in HDFS.

A *namespace* provides a logical grouping of tables. There are two predefined namespaces:

1. hbase — a system namespace, used to contain HBase internal tables

2. default — tables with no explicit specified namespace will automatically fall into this namespace

Users may define their own namespaces or may use the *default* namespace.

HBase Architecture

HBase has three major components:

1. A lightweight process, namely **HBase HMaster**, manages and monitors the Hadoop cluster, provides an interface for creating, updating, and deleting tables, and assigns regions to region servers in the Hadoop cluster for load balancing.

2. The **Region Servers** are the worker nodes in HBase. A region server runs on an HDFS DataNode and handles any 'read', 'write', 'update', and 'delete' request from the client. It has the following components: a *Block Cache* which stores the most frequently read data; a *MemStore* which stores new data that is not yet written to the disk; a *Write Ahead Log*, which is a file that stores new data that is not persisted to permanent storage; and the *HFile*, which is the actual storage file that stores the rows as sorted key values on a disk.

3. **ZooKeeper** for coordinating and monitoring the services.

HMaster and Region servers are registered with ZooKeeper. A client contacts the ZooKeeper in order to connect with region servers and HMaster.

Important Features of HBase

The particular features of HBase which make the data store efficient for certain kind of applications are as follows:

• Unlike Cassandra, HBase is not an 'eventually consistent' data store. Thus, it is suitable for the tasks requiring high consistency level.

• It supports automatic sharding, i.e., the regions can be split automatically and re-distributed when the data grows.

• Automatic RegionServer failover

- HBase uses HDFS as its underlying distributed file system.

- It can be easily integrated with Hadoop. MapReduce programs can be used to process HBase data and thus, massive parallel processing can be enabled.

- HBase supports Java API for data access, and also Thrift and REST services for non-Java front-ends.

- HBase supports Block Cache and Bloom Filters for query optimisation.

Further Reading

Tutorials on HBase and guidelines for efficient schema design may be found in [19] [7] [22] [12].

7.7   Graph Databases

Graph databases primarily emphasise on the relationships among the pieces of information. Thus, highly connected datasets can be easily stored in graph databases. In other types of databases, a complex query needs join of multiple tables or similar types of operations. On the other hand, complex queries can easily be executed on graph databases.

Graph databases are based on the *property graph model*. A property graph contains nodes connected through edges. *Nodes* represent entities and hold any number of attributes (key-value pairs) describing the entities. Nodes are sometimes assigned with labels, which define the role of the entities in the particular domain. In other words, labels help to place a set of nodes in one class.

On the other hand, edges represent relationships between the entities and hence are directed and named to represent semantically relevant connections between two entities. Like the nodes, relationships can also have properties. In general, these properties are some quantitative attributes, such as weight, cost, distance, etc. One such graph model is shown in Figure 7.6.

The following subsection describes Neo4j, one popular graph database.

7.7.1   Neo4j

Neo4j is one of the popular graph databases. It is based on the *property graph model* to store and manage the data.

Neo4j Data Model

The main building blocks of a graph database are *nodes*, *relationships* and *properties*. Each node in Neo4j represents an entity. Thus, nodes are the pri-

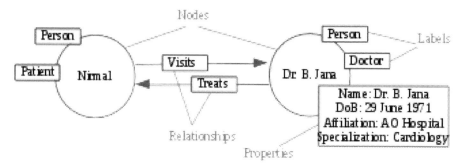

FIGURE 7.6: Property Graph Model

mary data elements. Nodes are described by properties, i.e. the attributes which are stored as key-value pairs. It is possible to define constraints for the properties. Indexes can also be created based on properties. Composite indexes can be created from multiple properties. The roles of a node in the graph are defined by labels. Neo4j allows the users to specify multiple labels for nodes. Labels are used to group nodes into sets.

Edges connecting two nodes in the graph represent relationships. Relationships are directional, i.e., the graph contains directed edges. Multiple relationships can be defined between two nodes. Like nodes, relationships can have one or more properties.

Neo4j Graph Platform

The Neo4j Graph Platform is shown in Figure 7.7. At the centre there exists the Neo4j graph database. The database supports transactional applications and graph analytics.

Specific features of Neo4j architecture are defined as follows:

- It maintains the ACID properties, i.e. 'Atomicity', 'Consistency', 'Isolation' and 'Durability'. In order to store an updated relationship between two nodes, simply writing a relationship record is not sufficient, but the node at each end of the relationship must be updated as well. If any one of these three write operations fails, it will result in a corrupted graph. To avoid creation of a corrupted graph, ACID properties are ensured in Neo4j.

- It allows the users to use flexible schema, i.e., the users can add or remove properties as and when the business requirement changes. Users can introduce or remove schema constraints for enterprise governance or rules enforcement.

- Integrity of the graph is assured by enforcing uniqueness of a node based on the combined uniqueness of a set of property values.

- It offers efficient and high performance query execution by allowing the user

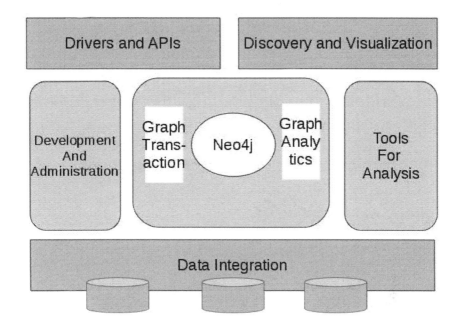

FIGURE 7.7: Neo4j Graph Platform [Source: [6]]

to search through the huge number of data connections in the graph. Each node directly references its adjacent nodes. Thus, there is no need for global indexes and the graph can be traversed in any direction using the graph nodes and relationships. The query time is proportional to the size of the graph searched and not the overall size of the data.

Neo4j Query Language

Cypher Query Language or CQL is used as the query language for Neo4j. CQL is a declarative pattern-matching language. It has a syntax similar to SQL.

Supporting Tools for Neo4j

The tools which are used for analysis and visualisation of data are as follows:

- Graph analytics: There are many graph algorithms which can traverse the graph efficiently. Neo4j graph algorithms, which are based on these algorithms, assist the users traverse the graph to read data from the nodes and analyse the data. The algorithms are available as an open procedure library. The library can be used by incorporating procedure calls in CQL.

- Graph visualisation: The Neo4j browser is a visualisation tool which helps creating the database and developing applications. Other tools which of-

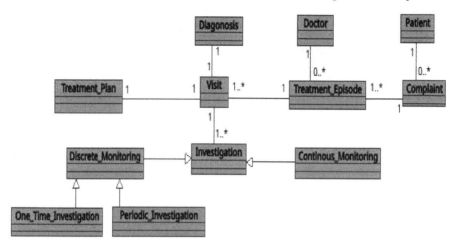

FIGURE 7.8: A hierarchical data model for health data

fer Neo4j graph visualisation include Tableu, Tom Sawyer, Linkurious, and Keylines.

Further Reading

Neo4j tutorials are available in [24] and [6].

7.8   Health Data Storage: A Case Study

We have made some study regarding how the health data can be stored in different storage systems and how different NoSQL databases behave when the health data are stored and retrieved from these databases [15][16]. While doing this study, in contrast to the flat data models proposed in several research articles, we used a hierarchical data model as shown in Figure 7.8.

In this data model, there may be multiple treatment episodes for a complaint (a complaint is related to a health problem of a patient for which the patient visits a doctor), and during a treatment episode, a patient may visit the doctor multiple times. The doctor may recommend certain medications in the treatment plan or ask for further investigations, such as pathological tests, monitoring of vitals, etc. While monitoring, data may be gathered from continuous monitoring, which will generate a time series data, or data may be of a discrete nature when it is collected at a particular time instant. Data from discrete monitoring is further subdivided into two categories: periodic (blood pressure measured every day) and one-time (e.g., X-ray, etc.). Sensor data may also be stored in this data model.

In this section, some experiences of storing the data in Cassandra are discussed. The key concept in Cassandra data modeling is denormalisation. One should plan in such a way that each query can be satisfied by one single column family. Thus denormalization can be used to increase read performance in Cassandra. The possible queries within the proposed framework must be first taken into consideration. Then the following steps can be followed:

- Step I: Important fields involving the common queries which are expected in the database are to be noted down.

- Step II: All fields are initially kept in one column family .

- Step III: A set of queries are considered and their execution statistics (for example, how many times such a query is run in real life and what are the performance requirements) are determined.

- Step IV: Mapping of the data model in the big data solution (here Cassandra) is determined in such a way that it will be appropriate for the specified queries to run. The queries must also run satisfying their performance requirement.

- Step V: Step IV is implemented by taking a single query and trying to find the best mapping in the big data solution. There might be a number of possible mapping proposals for each such query. It is a general practice to implement each accepted mapping and measure the performance of query execution, or to use a standard testing technique like YCSB (Yahoo! Cloud Serving Benchmark) [`https://s.yimg.com/ge/labs/v1/files/ycsb-v4.pdf`][5]. The proposal for a single query that performs best is selected.

- Step VI: Implementation is done in iterations and the mapped data model changes with every iteration. It is necessary to test, measure the performance and repeat the procedure for each such solution.

Since one of the main objectives for normalisation is to remove redundancies, denormalisation will actually lead to some redundancies. While designing the data model, it is also to be kept in mind that join operations are discouraged in big data solutions, as joining requires accessing multiple tables with huge data and results in high seek time.

There are few rules of thumb for designing a data model in Cassandra. The first one is that a proper row key should be chosen. Cassandra shows best performance when all the data required to answer a given query is located under the same partition key. The other thumb rule is that read-heavy data should be kept separate from write-heavy data.

The queries which have been considered while designing the Cassandra data model are as follows:

---

[5]YCSB is an open-source specification and program suite which is often used to evaluate retrieval and maintenance capabilities of computer programs.

1. Specialisation-wise doctor search (e.g., find all doctors' names and their details with specialization 'cardiologist').

2. Patient-wise information, like demographic information, food habits etc. (e.g., find the allergy details of patient having name 'Bijan Pal').

3. Organisation-wise doctor search (e.g., find the names of all doctors' who are attached to the organisation whose id is 'Apollo Hospital').

4. Patient-wise complaint search (e.g., find all complaint details of patient having the name 'Amit Chatterjee' between January 2017 and June 2018).

5. Complaint-wise treatment search (e.g., find all the treatment history for patient having the name 'Monica Bose' with complaint 'Headache').

Many database designers advise that if related data of a query is present in compact form in one column family in Cassandra, then its performance improves. However, it is practically impossible to create one single large table for all related information, and the performance cannot improve in such cases. Thus, we have taken an approach which will consider each query and propose a column family for that one although there will have been many iterations before arriving at a final solution. Thus, for queries 1 and 3, a **Doctor** column family containing fields like specialisation and organisation along with other basic details has been created. Likewise, all patient details are stored in the **Patient** column family.

The fourth query needs details of the patients' complaints along with some basic patient data. The fifth query requires that there must be a column family containing complaint details and details of investigations. It is evident that whenever there is a complaint, a treatment episode starts. Since Cassandra does not support joining of column families, simply storing the complaint_id along with the patient or treatment episode data (like a foreign key in relational databases) will not serve the purpose. Thus, the details of the complaint, investigations, etc., should be stored in one column family along with some details about the patient and the doctor. Considering all such facts, the patient has been divided into two parts — some basic information like demographic data, allergy details, food habits, etc., which are not likely to change much, is stored in the **Patient** column family. Another set of patient related fields which need continuous updating or writing and are necessary for understanding the complaint or to deal with medical investigations are separated and stored in a different column family. This column family is called **Treatment_Episode**. As a doctor is associated with each complaint of the illness of a patient, some necessary details of the doctors (such as doctor_id, name, and specialisation) are also stored in Treatment_Episode. Other than the information about the patient and the doctor, this column family stores the details of the complaint (symptoms, etc.), starting date of the treatment, the disease diagnosed, and the clinical status. A flag is stored to indicate whether the treatment is still active or not.

The next column family is a wide column family named **Visits**. This column family contains a visit_id unique to each visit of a patient to a doctor. It also contains information about the treatment, such as start date, initial complaint, patient and doctor details, and information about the visits, like date and time and reason for the visit. It includes clinical information like body temperature, pulse rate, height, weight, systolic and diastolic blood pressure, list of investigations prescribed by the doctor along with their reports as key-value pairs, medication prescribed along with rules as key-value pairs, diagnosis done by the doctor, therapies undergone, and current clinical status. Sensor data generated from continuous monitoring has been proposed to keep in a separate file. However, in the current study, sensor data has not been gathered and stored.

In Cassandra, it is possible to create a super column family, as discussed in Section 7.6.1. However, a super column family in this case requires many levels of nesting which decreases performance and is practically difficult to implement. Through our study, such degradation of performance has also been observed. A dynamic column family has a variable number of columns. It is also possible to create a dynamic column family by keeping complaint details including treatment and investigation details against a complaint_id. But some of the queries which have been considered in this study, particularly the simple queries do not perform well if a dynamic schema is used.

For three of the column families, composite keys have been created to improve the search performance. For the **Patient** column family, a simple primary key, *patient_id*, is used for searching. For the three other column families, the first field of the composite key is chosen in such a way that it decides the order of searching. The data related to the similar values of the first attribute are stored in one partition. For example, for both column families, **Treatment_Episode** and **Visits**, *patient_id* is chosen as the first field of the composite key. This allows all records related to a single patient to be stored in one partition, thus reducing communication costs across the computing nodes storing different partitions. The composite row key of **Treatment_Episode** is chosen as *(patient_id, doctor_id , treatment_id)* and the composite row key of **Visits** is chosen as *(patient_id, treatment_id, visit_id)*. There is one single entry for each doctor in the **Doctor** column family. Therefore, for this column family, *(specialisation, doctor_id)* has been chosen as the row key, and thus, the doctor records are partitioned based on the specialisation. Such an arrangement is effective for the the second query in our list [15].

Indexes may be used for a column family when it is used for a single query. But an index may not be efficient to perform different types of queries on one column family. Indexes have not been used in this study.

7.9 Chapter Notes

This chapter discusses different solutions for storing and managing big data. It is well understood that unstructured and semi-structured data generated through various healthcare applications cannot be stored in relational databases because of their rigid structure. Therefore, NoSQL databases have been introduced, and many healthcare application developers are currently inclined to use these databases. However, there are many different types of NoSQL databases, including key-value stores, document databases, column-oriented databases, graph databases etc. The architecture, data model, partitioning and data distribution philosophy, and implementation of read-write operations are different in these databases. Nevertheless, many of these databases have interesting features which are effective for managing big data.

The chapter reviews some of the NoSQL database solutions and indicates the important properties of each. Finally, the chapter presents a case study of storing health data using one of the popular big data solutions, namely Cassandra. Although, the study involves only a single database, it provides some insights about how one should approach the problem of storing health data.

References

[1] Apache Cassandra. Website: https://cassandra.apache.org/.

[2] Apache CouchDB. Website: http://docs.couchdb.org/en/2.1.1/intro/index.html.

[3] Data Management for Cloud Applications: DataStax. Website: http://www.datastax.com/.

[4] MongoDB Manual. Website: https://docs.mongodb.com/manual/.

[5] MongoDB Tutorial for Beginners. Website: https://www.guru99.com/mongodb-tutorials.html.

[6] The Internet–Scale Graph Platform. Website: https://neo4j.com/, 2016.

[7] Overview of hbase architecture and its components. Website: https://www.dezyre.com/article/overview-of-hbase-architecture-and-its-components/295, 2016.

[8] M. Allen. 5 Reasons – RDBMS Aren't Working. Website: http://www.marklogic.com/blog/relational-databases-change/.

[9] F. Chang, J. Dean, S. Ghemawat, W. C. Hsieh, D. A. Wallach, M. Burrows, T. Chandra, A. Fikes, and R. E. Gruber. Bigtable: A distributed storage system for structured data. *ACM Transactions on Computer Systems (TOCS)*, 26(2):4, 2008.

[10] S. Grimes. Unstructured Data and the 80 Percent Rule. Website: https://breakthroughanalysis.com/2008/08/01/unstructured-data-and-the-80-percent-rule/, August 2008.

[11] A. Haseeb and G. Pattun. A review on NoSQL: Applications and challenges. *International Journal of Advanced Research in Computer Science*, 8(1), 2017.

[12] A. Khurana. Introduction to HBase Schema Design. *White Paper, Cloudera*, 2012.

[13] A. Mehra. Introduction to Apache Cassandra's Architecture. Website: https://dzone.com/articles/introduction-apache-cassandras, 2015.

[14] M. Mulcahy. Big Data Are You in Control? Website: `https://www.waterfordtechnologies.com/big-data-interesting-facts/`, February 2017.

[15] K. Naguri, P. Sil Sen, and N. Mukherjee. Design of a health-data model and a query-driven implementation in Cassandra. In *E-health Networking, Application & Services (HealthCom), 2015 17th International Conference on*, pages 144–148. IEEE, 2015.

[16] H. S. Ray, K. Naguri, P. Sil Sen, and N. Mukherjee. Comparative Study of Query Performance in a Remote Health Framework using Cassandra and Hadoop. In *Proceedings of the 9th International Joint Conference on Biomedical Engineering Systems and Technologies (BIOSTEC 2016)– Volume 5: HEALTHINF, Rome, Italy, February 21–23, 2016*, pages 330–337, 2016.

[17] Sherpa Software. Structured and Unstructured Data: What is It? Website: `https://sherpasoftware.com/blog/structured-and-unstructured-data-what-is-it/`.

[18] C. Strozzi. NoSQL: a non-SQL RDBMS. Website: `http://www.strozzi.it/cgi-bin/CSA/tw7/I/en\_US/NoSQL/Home%20Page`.

[19] Apache HBase Team. Apache HBase Reference Guide. Website: `http://hbase.apache.org/book.html\#conceptual.view`.

[20] Tutorialspoint. Cassandra Tutorial. Website: `https://www.tutorialspoint.com/cassandra/index.htm`.

[21] Tutorialspoint. CouchDB Tutorial. Website: `https://www.tutorialspoint.com/couchdb/couchdb\_attaching\_files.htm`.

[22] Tutorialspoint. HBase Tutorial. Website: `https://www.tutorialspoint.com/hbase/index.htm`.

[23] Tutorialspoint. MongoDB Tutorial. Website: `https://www.tutorialspoint.com/mongodb/mongodb\_indexing.htm`.

[24] Tutorialspoint. Neo4j Tutorial. Website: `https://www.tutorialspoint.com/hbase/index.htm`.

8

Security and Privacy for Health Data

CONTENTS

8.1	Introduction	....	192
	8.1.1	Security	....	192
	8.1.2	Privacy	....	193
	8.1.3	Privacy-Preserving Data Management	....	194
	8.1.4	A Few Common Questions	....	197
8.2	Security and Privacy Issues	....	198
	8.2.1	Storage	....	199
	8.2.2	Security Breach	....	199
	8.2.3	Data Mingling	....	200
	8.2.4	Data Sensitivity	....	200
	8.2.5	User	....	202
	8.2.6	Computations	....	202
	8.2.7	Transaction Logs	....	202
	8.2.8	Validation of Input	....	202
	8.2.9	Data Mining	....	203
	8.2.10	Access Control	....	203
	8.2.11	Data Audit	....	204
	8.2.12	Data Source	....	205
	8.2.13	Security Best Practices	....	206
	8.2.14	Software Security	....	207
	8.2.15	Secure Hardware	....	207
	8.2.16	User Account Management	....	207
	8.2.17	Clustering and Auditing of Databases	....	208
8.3	Challenges	....	208
	8.3.1	Malicious User	....	208
	8.3.2	Identifying Threats	....	209
	8.3.3	Risk Mitigation	....	209
	8.3.4	Real-Time Monitoring	....	210
	8.3.5	Privacy Preservation	....	210
		8.3.5.1	Health Data Sale	....	212
		8.3.5.2	Compliance for EHR	....	212
8.4	Security of NoSQL Databases	....	213
	8.4.1	Reviewing Security in NoSQL databases	....	213
		8.4.1.1	Security in Cassandra	....	214

          8.4.1.2   Security in MongoDB 215
          8.4.1.3   Security in HBase 216
      8.4.2   Reviewing Enterprise Approaches towards Security in
               NoSQL Databases 218
8.5   Integrating Security with Big Data Solutions 219
      8.5.1   Big Data Enterprise Security 220
8.6   Secured Health Data Delivery: A Case Study 223
8.7   Chapter Notes 227

8.1 Introduction

Nowadays, data represents an important asset. Regardless of the backgrounds they are coming from, data tries to contribute something to the applications they are used for. So what we see is that an increasing number of organisations collect data, very often concerning individuals. This is then used for a variety of purposes ranging from scientific research, as in the case of medical data, to demographic trend analysis and marketing. Due to different reasons, organisations may also sometimes give access to the data owned by them to third parties. This widely available data therefore poses threats to the security and privacy of individuals and organisations.

8.1.1 Security

Security is the prevention of, or protection against, unauthorised access to information and/or resources, and intentional and unauthorised destruction or alteration of information [4]. It can therefore be said from the above definition that appropriate measures for stopping unauthorszed access is security. This also means that measures adopted for defending any information and/or resource is security. Sometimes this unauthorised access may be utilised for destruction, or alteration and hence it becomes a deliberate action. Security is considered to have three aspects [4]: Confidentiality, Integrity, and Availability.

1. Confidentiality is defined as protection against unauthorised disclosure. Let X be a set of entities and let I be some information. I is said to have the property of confidentiality with respect to X if no member of X can obtain information about I.

2. Integrity is defined as the protection of information against unauthorised modification. This is generally called *data* integrity. Integrity may be defined for the source or generator of information. Protection of the validity of the source is *source* integrity. Let X be a set of entities and let I be some information or a resource. I is said to have the property of integrity with respect to X if all members of

X validate I by some validation method or all members of X trust I as they validate the source of I by some authentication process.

3. Availability is defined as the property of a system to always be present to meet requirements. Let X be a set of entities and let I be a resource. I is said to have the property of availability with respect to X if all members of X can access I whenever the requirement arises.

8.1.2 Privacy

Privacy is defined to be the state in which one does not want to be observed or does not want any attention, as if existence is away from public notice or attention. But all the while, existence is present. This makes the existence itself opaque. The term *privacy* seems to supplement *security*. As observed in 8.1.1, providing *confidentiality* aspects to resource or information would keep prying eyes away from it. Any unauthorised usage will not be able to get through it. As an example: Suppose an encoded message reaches an unauthorised user. He will not be able to decode the message and unearth the true meaning until and unless he knows the proper method to decode the message. Thus, the message exists, and can also be seen, but cannot be deciphered. In our daily life though we tend to use the terms confidentiality and privacy interchangeably, these are definitely distinct from a legal standpoint. With respect to healthcare, confidentiality refers to personal health information shared with one's physician. The relationship between a doctor and his patient implies confidentiality since the doctor is going to help the patient by analysing his health information. However, this health-related medical information is considered to be *private* information of the patient. The doctor is not supposed to reveal this private information to all and sundry. But the pharmacist may know or guess the patient's health condition by looking into the medicines that the doctor has prescribed for this patient. Apart from the doctor, the patient has the right to use his private information.

It is to be noted here that the doctor has not breached the *confidentiality* pact, since it is his primary duty to prescribe for the patient. But any other action taken by the doctor may be considered to be a breach. Thus, health information of a patient can be kept encoded and the access may be limited to the patient and his doctor, and some special user. So, *privacy* of information can be achieved through methods that are adopted for *confidentiality*.

In a nutshell, with reference to healthcare, *privacy* is considered to be the right of an individual to keep his health information private, whereas *confidentiality* is the duty of the person entrusted with that health information to keep that information private and not make the information available to the public.

The simplest concern about privacy is that information must not be revealed. This also depends on the requirements of the application. There may be serious consequences if privacy is not maintained. For example, the name of a disease along with the name of the patient reveal that the patient is suffering from that disease. If the disease comes with a some sort of social stigma in a particular society, then the revelation may make the suffering worse for the patient. The patient will be getting treatment, but other societal norms and pressures may not be beneficial for his health. An interesting fact that is coming up from the example is that there is another concern regarding privacy. The association of the disease name and patient name puts the well being of the patient at risk, since it comes out in the open that the patient is suffering from that disease. It is, however, not necessary for everybody to know the exact disease the patient is suffering from. The doctor treating the patient, and the associates at the health clinic or hospital, may know the identity of the patient and the disease. Hence, only the persons who need to know the association (between the patient and the disease) should be aware of this association. Hence, this association too needs to be guarded.

For some different applications, information about the disease and information about the patient may be needed but in entirely different contexts. This means that the situation in which the disease name will be needed will not require the patient's name. So the information will be used separately where there is no need for the association. This implies that the information may therefore exist separately and be available (whenever necessary) accordingly. But in the other context, proper measures have to be taken to link these two different pieces of information (patient name, disease name) in such a way that it is invisible to the outside world. Any intentional approach to discover the linkage will then be thwarted. So this association needs privacy. It is also now apparent from the above discussion that *confidentiality* alone may not be able to provide the required *privacy*.

8.1.3   Privacy-Preserving Data Management

As evident from the above discussions, privacy has become a great concern to both users and organisations. The main issue becomes data management. Since data generally belongs to an individual, it is important to handle it carefully and according to application requirements. Therefore, research efforts are also making their presence known in handling data privacy related issues. The *Privacy-Preserving* data-management technique is one such development [2].

Data is sometimes released to third parties by data owners. Since data once released is not under the control of the organisations owning it, they are unable to control how the data will be used. One of the simplest techniques can be to modify the data in such a way that no information that can directly link data items with individuals still remains in the data. This process is referred to as *data anonymisation* . However, easier said than done! This process of simply deleting information like name or phone number or address in the released data may not be enough. Some hitherto unknown links may exist. It is experimentally shown that even when such information is removed, it may still be possible to link the remaining data with other information. This combination can reveal the individual this data refers to.

The work in [38] proposed approaches based on the notion of *k-anonymity* . Suppose a data holder wants to share or release a part of its data with one particular category of users. The challenge is to ensure that the subjects of the data are not re-identified with this sharing. The author proposed a formal protection model, named *k-anonymity*, along with a set of policies. A release of the data will provide *k-anonymity* protection if information for each subject in the release is indistinguishable from at least k-1 subjects whose information is also contained in the same release.

Privacy-preservation in the context of data mining is also important. Several approaches for specific data mining techniques, like tools for association rule mining or classification systems, and others that are independent of any specific data mining technique, are found in literature. Generally, all of these techniques are based on modification of data. Modification may be the only way of reducing the confidence of sensitive association rules as found in techniques specialised for privacy-preserving mining of association rules. However with data undergoing too many modifications, the resultant database may not be qualified for use.

Techniques are also proposed and developed that estimate errors cropping up due to modifications in the database. This estimation may be used to have a check on how the modification would be done. Techniques are also developed based on *commutative encryption,* which supports distributed data mining processes on encrypted data [7]. The technique deals with data at multiple sites. The algorithms running on these sites share some information to calculate results. It is also shown that the shared information does not disclose private data.

Research efforts are also noticed in designing Database Management Systems (DBMS) specifically supporting privacy policies. The authors in [30] presented the concept of Hippocratic databases that incorporate privacy protection in relational database systems. The database architecture incorporates features that use some privacy metadata consisting of privacy policies and privacy authorisations. These are stored in privacy-policies tables and privacy-authorisations tables, respectively. However, there is still demand for more. The development of such database technology will have to address a lot of challenging issues ranging from modeling to architectures. This may eventually lead to the next-generation of DBMS.

Privacy has to be enforced once data collection is done, since data will most likely be stored using some DBMS. Hence, developing DBMS that can enforce privacy promises and other privacy policies is crucial. Privacy-preserving DBMS pose several challenges to both theory and architecture. It seems that tools for data anonymisation and privacy-preserving data mining may be required for developing *privacy-preserving* DBMS.

In general, *privacy-preserving* DBMS must provide support for privacy-specific metadata. This may be associated with the data and can be stored in the database together with the data. The requirement may be that a specific metadata can be associated with an entire table, with a single tuple, or even with a column within a single tuple, in a relational database management system.

The well-known Role-Based Access Control (RBAC) model is generally provided in DBMS. There is hardly any scope of specifying application-dependent user profiles that can be used for access control and privacy enforcement. The specification of application-dependent user profiles may be supported as extensions of RBAC models [7].

In the context of privacy, obligations play an important role in specifying privacy-related actions on data access for certain purposes. Trigger mechanisms, available in all commercial DBMS, are able to manage the privacy-related actions on data access.

Fine-grained access control always seems to be one of the most important requirements. It is also important to maintain privacy policy even if data flows across domains or systems. Though some of these properties may already be supported by existing DBMS, they may require insightful details for preserving privacy.

The authors in [2] pointed out that to provide privacy-protecting access control, the purpose for which access is required may be taken into account. The approach is based on finding the intended purposes, since these specify the intended usage of data, and access purposes. The authors also introduce the notion of purpose compliance, which forms the basis for verifying the purpose of the data access. The work also addresses data labeling schemes, which is association of data with intended purposes. Granularity of data labeling is considered here with respect to relational databases.

But how will a system determine the purpose of an access request? The above mentioned work makes it simple by taking the information (what is the purpose for the request?) from the users themselves. The request would be validated and then the request is executed. Data labeling may specify the purpose for which the data is to be accessed. This labeling may be carried on for each data attribute of a data element. Suppose a record contains name, age, height, weight, and address attributes. Labeling may be done depending upon the application requirement. For example, with phone number, if the label is *not to be accessed for marketing or advertisement purposes*, and if the request says, 'find phone number for tax form', the purpose of the request is clear and validated and hence access will be granted. The authors also modified queries for access control. Suppose there is a query for name and phone number for marketing purposes. The query result would provide only the name and not the phone number. In this work [2], *role-based access control* is used with *attribute-based access control.*

However, the development of such a model that incorporates all privacy-preserving issues is a hard one.

8.1.4   A Few Common Questions

Up until now, people (developers and users alike) were hardly aware of the fact that big data from an application is generally stored or saved in some storage which may not be exclusively owned by the developer or the system that is generating the data. Storage systems based on cloud are the best alternative storage option as of now. We have already talked about this in Chapter 3. However, this has given rise to an entire range of questions in the minds of the various stakeholders of the system. We are going to discuss a few of them here.

One of the questions is: 'Who is accessing my data?' Of course, it is only the application developers and the users whom they authorise who will be able to access the data. But since the data is not stored within the physical premises of the organisation, everybody gets worried. Hence there is need for discussion, particularly about access control practices.

Another question goes like: 'Which data is being accessed?' This, in reality, means: Is the entire database or some of the data files being accessed? It is not apparent how it will matter if we happen to know which data is accessed. We shall not be able to delete this data from the accessor's log. Actually, the main concern with this question is, whether it is *my* data file or file of somebody else's. I may not be bothered if the file belongs to somebody else.

'When was the access?' is another common question. This is like: Had we known earlier, we could have taken some measures and avoided it!! So, why not take the measure at the very beginning?

Some may also ask 'Where is the access from?' People want to know the answer to this question, so that they could identify the threat point and may try to avoid this point in future. It may not occur to them that it is not always easy to identify the threat points in the vast network. The actual attack surface may be large.

Questions like: 'Is there a data breach?' have also come up. Everybody thinks that since he cannot physically keep the data, all accesses are unauthorised accesses. It may not occur to the users that data access is also provided in a thoughtful manner. Data breach, after all, may not occur, at all.

Not everyone is concerned with compliance, but in such situations, people will ask: 'Is there a breach in compliance?' This is asked as if all blame may be put on the organisation for non-compliance.

People are mostly concerned about: 'How will we know what is happening?' These same people may never be bothered about what was happening when data was kept with them, but now that the data is outside of the organisation, they feel concerned. They always want to know whether someone is looking into their data or guarding their data, because otherwise there is no way of knowing what is happening with their data. However, the concern should be the same as when data was with them.

'Are we under attack?' is a very common question. This question comes from lack of awareness. Many people do not have any idea about *attack*, and hence, whenever some incident occurs, they think *attack* is underway. They are unable to distinguish between *threat* and *attack*. Awareness is the only key here.

The next couple of sections discuss the issues and possible measures for security and privacy.

8.2   Security and Privacy Issues

Big health data brings with itself big security problems [10]. As already discussed in the previous section, health data not only needs to be secured but also needs privacy. The big security problems are mainly due to the variety and velocity of the data, along with other things. There is little time to handle the various changing forms of data. The data's being voluminous is also of great concern. As soon as the data of a certain instant is secured, data of the next instant arrives and demands immediate attention. Hence, a number of issues crop up. These issues need to be addressed properly in order to obtain a secure health system.

8.2.1   Storage

The data is generally kept in cloud servers and hence not in centralised storage. The data is actually spread over a number of storage servers and needs to be retrieved carefully. Since a query may be related to any data, more than one server may have to be involved in answering the query. This requires the servers to be always available, leading to the reliability issue. The servers deployed to store the data must be functional so that the query is handled appropriately. To achieve high reliability, issues related to failure detection, failure rate, and recovery time may be studied. Since health data is crucial for the well being of a patient, measures of fault tolerance may be taken. The simplest may be replication of data in replica servers, a method widely practised in distributed systems. However, this will increase the overhead, as data stored in all replicas has to be secured and synchronised any time data is being added, modified, or deleted. Thus, the issue of non-centralised storage must also address the issues of availability and reliability.

8.2.2   Security Breach

A security breach is said to occur when a system experiences unauthorised access. If such unauthorised access is not detected and therefore continues, the system may be beyond authorised control. Effectively, the system will be unavailable to valid users in no time. So, a security breach has to be addressed as being of the utmost importance. Measures against breaches have to be aimed towards user authentication and access control. This will prevent the system from being usurped by unauthorised access, leading to unavailability. Implementation of proper authentication and access control mechanisms will take care of users and accidental access, among other things.

In particular, data breaches in healthcare applications may occur from various interaction points. In fact, data breaches are common phenomena in healthcare industries. These not only become expensive to deal with but also leave the system and its users at loggerheads, since users are unable to rely on the system. Each of them will be blaming the other. The cases of data breach may range from stealing protected health information to committing medical identity theft, implying that an unauthorised person gets access to medical records of a patient when he is not authorised to do so. Motives and outcomes notwithstanding, the incidents prove costly to be fought out.

Generally, several factors are found to be responsible for data breaches. Apart from unauthorised access, data may be lost due to negligence or other causes, or worse: data theft may occur. Another often overlooked cause is the way data are disposed off. Whenever there is no need for some data, it is our tendency to just either delete it or put it in some storage media and not look back. But some malicious user may be present in the system, someone who is more than happy to take care of this data!

Thus, healthcare organisations, hospitals, and associated industries including medical device manufacturers need to be careful about protecting sensitive patient, financial, and other data as well as device-specific information.

8.2.3 Data Mingling

Data will be stored in a cloud environment where data from many other applications will also be stored. Thus, data from more than one unrelated application will be stored together. Hence, access to data will also be from different unrelated applications. If proper measures are not adopted, unauthorised access may take place. The responsibility also lies with the cloud service provider in separating out each data source and treating each of them individually. However, the applications themselves should also take care to avoid unauthorised access. To be fair, both parties (data owners and storage providers) must be aware of their responsibilities.

Cloud service providers may be located in countries other than that of the customers. Hence, laws governing data may differ across geographic boundaries. The laws of one's own nation may not be applicable if the data is not located in that nation. The situation may also be such that data is located in a country which enforces strict laws, but the data actually might be stored physically within a database elsewhere. In the database, the data is likely to co-exist with other data from a number of different companies and organisations, probably from different countries. The data will be protected by strict cyber security laws, but the co-mingling cannot be avoided.

The responsibility, therefore, lies with all stakeholders to keep data safe and sound, in spite of the situations described above.

8.2.4 Data Sensitivity

We are talking here about healthcare applications for data. It is well known that data related to health is always sensitive. However, health data may still be classified under different categories with respect to sensitivity. Not all data is sensitive, per se. And some information is absolutely necessary for keeping the entire record related to the patient. In the patient's health record there will be demographic information of the patient, his vitals (like height, weight, age), the symptoms he has come down with, and finally, the possible diagnosis, prescribed medicines or medical tests, or both tests and diagnosis, as deemed necessary by the doctor. This patient record is likely to be modified each time a patient visits the doctor. It may so happen that information from among these different information fields (of the patient record) gets revealed. This revelation may not always pose a privacy risk. But if the revealed information is that patient *P1* has disease *D1*, then this is a sensitive information with respect to *P1*. Hence, this information must not be disclosed. However, for some other disease *D2*, and patient *P2* having that disease *D2* may not be as sensitive as the former. This may depend on the social stigma attached to *D1* and *D2*. So, this information (*P2* and *D2*) may be disclosed. Many a time, medical test results may reveal information that the patient does not want to disclose. A patient may be too sensitive to reveal his condition even if he is only advised to go for that test. On some other occasions, past health information of a patient or his relatives may also be a sensitive issue. Thus, the overall situation is sensitive, and hence, some individual data and combinations or groups of data have to be identified and categorised accordingly. This is required, to distinguish health data based on sensitivity. This task is complex, as domain expertise is needed.

One of the much-talked-about categories of sensitive information is *Personally Identifiable Information* (PII). This is associated with an individual person, such as an employee, student, or donor. The PII itself must be stored carefully and handled all the more carefully. Obviously, PII must not be accessed by all, and therefore, should have restricted access. PII should only be accessed when required on a strictly need-to-know basis. Needless to say, PII has to be handled and stored with care. This is because, PII is the only information that can be used to uniquely identify, contact, or locate a single person.

For example, the following individually identifiable data fields, when combined in a specific fashion, will be able to reveal personal health information.

1. Name
2. Telephone numbers
3. Email addresses
4. Social Security number (countries other than India) or Aadhaar number (India)
5. Medical Record number
6. Health Insurance Plan number
7. License Plate numbers
8. Full-face Photographic images
9. Thumb Impression

The Medical Record number assumes that EHR is followed. The above list is not exhaustive, but it may be a pointer as to how sensitive patient health information may be identified.

8.2.5   User

Proper authentication mechanism will allow valid users into the system. Generally, we tend to put our faith in the users. However, a valid and authenticated user may turn malicious with time. Hence, the most important consideration will be to not implicitly *trust* any user. Handling of this issue therefore needs a bigger picture, where it can be ascertained whether a user can be *trusted* or not. This is, rather, an issue with greater implications. The authenticated user may be doing activities that seem innocuous, at first. But his actions may affect places it is not supposed to affect. Hence, activities of a user in the system need to be followed. So, with all-out efforts, such users have to be reigned in at all times.

8.2.6   Computations

The framework for storage and computation is essentially distributed in nature. Hence, one of the main concerns is to ensure that computations are not done in the open; that is, so they cannot be viewed from anywhere in the system. This implies that computations must be done with proper security and under proper control. It may so happen that parameters for some computations may have to be sourced from various sites. The result may also have to be shipped to some other site. The system being distributed in nature, all information is mainly local and exchange of parameters or results or both have to be done securely, keeping *confidentiality* and *integrity* in mind. So, computations are to be performed maintaining security and in a secure environment.

8.2.7   Transaction Logs

As is well known, transaction logs behave like a faithful old-world recording system within a system. Transaction logs generally record details of the different events occurring in the system. So, this log is always a vital source of information to attackers for identifying the vulnerable points in the system. Hence, transaction logs have to handled with the utmost care, and the log must be guarded against access by unauthorized users. This will protect the log from mishandling (being used for ulterior purposes). Apart from that, the transaction log must be protected from tampering even by authenticated and authorised users. Many times, this may happen quite unintentionally. So, transaction logs may also be saved securely in some particular location in the system at regular intervals. This may prevent accidental access of the same.

8.2.8   Validation of Input

We are talking about healthcare systems which will generate big data, in every sense of the term. The data will be generated at various sources that may include: health centres, health kiosks, hospitals, pathological labs, body sensors, and so on. We may have a list of authorised health centres and hospitals, to start with. We can assume that data coming from these sources is genuine. However, with time this list will definitely grow but may shrink at certain places. It is very important to take note of the shrinkage, since data from that source will not be valid any more. This is just a simple example.

Many times, instruments may not be well calibrated, or there may be some other errors, or these may be mishandled. So, these instruments may give erroneous readings. Proper mechanisms must be in place to identify such outlier data, otherwise the diagnosis will be incorrect. An incorrect diagnosis may have innumerable effects, including fatality.

Still, there may be situations when data from body sensors arrives out of sequence or is delayed. Freshness of data may be an issue for continuous monitoring of patients. Hence, even if the cause of delay or other discrepancies cannot be determined in real-time, measures must be taken for detecting such anomalies and rectifying them.

8.2.9 Data Mining

There may not be any single, central storage space for data. As perceived and mentioned earlier, data may be distributed over numerous storage spaces across the network. User queries may come from any location and for any data, as well. It is required to get the result of the query within a reasonable time. Even after getting the results back, additional time would be required to make the result *effective*. This also depends on the query extraction method used. With data mining as the objective, queries have to be directed towards the corresponding objective. For example, a pharmacist wants to know whether there is any market for a drug that treats only a particular disease. The query first must satisfy this objective; that is, the query has to be built for getting information about the disease in a particular geographical region where the pharmacist is located or in which he is interested. It may not help if the query results produce thousands of regions where the disease is prevalent, because then a secondary query may have to be made for getting results related to the specific regions. Hence, it is apparent that effective results and extraction of meaning from those results will be hard to collate, given the nature of the query and the time of evaluation.

8.2.10 Access Control

Access Control issues have evolved with the evolution of computing paradigms. In a distributed and cloud environment, access control has become all the more complex. Another parameter that affects access control with respect to the current application of healthcare is privacy preservation. In this application, access to users has to be permitted very judiciously. The situation may be such that access once given may be revoked, too, whereas access once not provided may be provided in the future. Dynamic access control features may be required for healthcare applications hosted in the cloud.

Discretionary Access Control (DAC) is one of the most well-known access control model in which the data owner decides who will get what type of access to the data it owns. The other well-known approach is *Mandatory Access Control (MAC)*, in which the operating system has control over access to data by users.

One of the simplistic approaches would be *Role-Based Access Control (RBAC)*. It is assumed here that the users in a system are assigned predefined *roles*, probably based on the activities they perform in the system. In a healthcare application, the medical practitioner is assigned the role of *doctor*, the caregiver is assigned the role of *nurse*. Similarly, there are *patients*, *pharmacists*, and so on. These *roles* then become their identities in the system. Each role carries a set of privileges associated with it. This enables a user to have some specific *control* over system objects, based on these *roles*. Hence a doctor is able to read and write prescriptions, among many other tasks in the system, whereas a nurse or pharmacist will be able to read the prescription but never be allowed to write a prescription. This is one of the simplest examples of *role-based access*.

Attribute-based Access Control is another prevalent access control paradigm that assigns access rights to users based on policies combining attributes. The policy can use any type of attribute, user attribute, resource attribute, environment or contextual attribute, and so on. For example, say a doctor has prescribed a medicine to a patient based on his pathological report. If the actual medicine is not available, then the pharmacist may be allowed to *read* the pathological report and the symptoms, so that he can get an equivalent medicine. Otherwise, the pathologist is never allowed to read the pathological report. However, based on the contextual attribute that the prescribed medicine is not available, a policy may dictate that the pharmacist can *read* the pathological report.

8.2.11 Data Audit

An audit is the official inspection of the accounts an organisation holds. While extending the meaning of *audit* to data audit, it therefore means that an organisation similarly needs to periodically check its data. An audit is generally performed by an independent or third party. The same applies here, too.

Data needs to be audited to find and assess its suitability for the purpose. Metrics have to be drawn specifically for this purpose. An organisation may be the owner or user or both of a large amount of data. But that data may not be particularly useful to it, while the company has already been using it for quite some time. Hence, a data audit would be able to find out where and how the data resides, for what purposes it is being used, and likewise. This is how a data audit may be performed. However, the granularity, as to at which micro level the audit will be performed, remains a question. Likewise, whether the audit will be limited to data files or organisation of the data, or even different fields or attributes of the data!

8.2.12 Data Source

As is well known, big data is generated from varied sources, and in different formats, too. For a particular application, therefore, it will be helpful if designers, or developers, or users can pre-identify the data sources. This is one of the ways of identifying data sources. Knowing data sources beforehand will help application developers check the authenticity of the sources even before the application is deployed.

However, as the application runs, with time and demands from the application, other sources of data (not pre-identified) may seem to be useful. These data sources, will need particularly rigorous authentication. One major cause of concern is that these data sources may be well known and valid, but the requirement of including them as data sources in that particular application may be questionable.

It is really fascinating to see the ways in which health information may be gathered. For example, say a person P may casually mention that he has been running a fever for a couple of days. With all the other information of P already available (mostly online), inference about his health can be drawn almost immediately. If required, warnings may even be sounded to the appropriate authorities!! All of these things may not always have the approval of the person P, although it seems appropriate to have *his* permission first.

Prominent IT giants like IBM [14] and Symantech [39] have their own methodology for authentication of data sources. They integrated the methods in the respective data source templates. In hospital-based or health-centre-based healthcare applications, data sources will be pre-identified and hence authentication will be no big deal. But with other healthcare applications, including remote patient monitoring and patients with WBAN, data sources may vary with time. A patient will be attached to different devices for the purpose of continuous monitoring. Nevertheless, if the source is identified, some authentication can be sought by the application and, given the circumstances, the source may be authenticated.

8.2.13   Security Best Practices

Security best practices must be followed in any application that demands security, even if at the basic level. This is to be done as a measure for standardisation of applications. In healthcare applications, data being of different formats and sizes, best practices should be interwoven into the design and architecture of the application software, databases, and storages. A few directions towards prevalent best practices are mentioned below [24].

There are various ways by which a hacker or malicious user may break into healthcare data. It is seen that most firms spend money on perimeter security like firewalls and antivirus software. But experts are of the opinion that technologies should also be in place to limit the damage when attacks really occur. One possibility in such a scenario is network segregation. This will contain the intruder within one part of the network and the intruder's hand will not be extended beyond this part or region of the network.

Any IT security program must focus on training the employee. The employee must have lessons in various types of attacks, and how they should protect themselves from becoming targets of such attacks, or unknowingly becoming a partner in the crime. Simple advice on choice of passwords may also be provided.

A number of healthcare applications may store data on smart and mobile devices, even if temporarily. These data must be held in encrypted portable devices, and associated workers may be warned against carrying unencrypted devices. It may be advisable to use some sort of *mobile device management* on top of anti-malware software that is able to filter malicious input, by statistical similarity detection and outlier detection techniques.

It is a known fact that wireless networks are more prone to security threats. So, care has to be taken to secure the wireless network and the components. To protect against attacks, organisations have to keep routers and access points and other components of the wireless network up to date. Relevant passwords must be changed regularly and frequently, and unauthorised devices should be barred from accessing the network.

Although health data is kept electronically in most organisations, including hospitals and healthcare centres, a lot of information may still be on paper. In such cases, files have to be protected from unauthorised physical access.

It is high time that healthcare organisations framed policies on the usage of portable devices. The policy may state what types of applications and what types of data can be stored on what gadgets, and the time limit for storing them on these devices.

One of the practices that organisations should learn to use is deletion of unnecessary data. Healthcare organisations do not usually follow this practice. But the more data someone keeps, the greater is the probability of that data getting *leaked*. So, why take unnecessary risks? It therefore seems better not to keep patient information and data beyond a certain time!

Since security threats may arise from in-house users, it is important to monitor their access. It may be hard to detect whether the users have malicious intentions. The same is true for third parties, such as business partners, contractors, and vendors who have access to data. Their access must also be monitored.

Authentication mechanisms may include multi-factor authentication. Passwords must be changed regularly and default passwords should never be used.

It is not possible for an organisation to be able to prevent every possible IT security incident. Hence it is very important to develop a plan of action when a breach occurs.

8.2.14   Software Security

An important issue that always comes up is the platform and software referred to and used by designers and developers. Nowadays there are various platforms and software offering similar services. Developers have to be cautious enough to choose from these offerings and go for rather well-known secured platforms. Sometimes service from not-so-well-known source may be equally competitive, and the developer then has to devise some methodology for establishing the authenticity of that service before using it.

8.2.15   Secure Hardware

The hardware required to build the system should also be secured and kept protected. The stakeholders of the system may not have direct control over the hardware if cloud-based storage and computing are used. However, care must be taken during identifying such server units, depending upon the security policy and technique the provider is offering.

8.2.16   User Account Management

Managing user accounts may have some characteristics in common with user access control management. But even after providing a user with certain access, there is always a need for supervision to find out whether or not a user is misusing his rights. It is a known fact that many security attacks are launched by insiders only. Hence care has to be taken to find out the pattern of how a user makes use of an account. Warning messages may be produced or an alert may be sounded to administrators in the event of deviations. An idle user account is also to be probed. All of these activities can be monitored if a proper log is maintained and reviewed regularly.

8.2.17   Clustering and Auditing of Databases

For keeping this large amount of ever-growing data, different databases are required. These databases need to be clustered and stored. The decision of clustering has to consider certain parameters so that clustering and monitoring the health of the clusters is simple and causes low overhead. Regular auditing is also necessary to detect abnormalities in clustering and storage.

The issues identified above may be few, and among many others. But these above-mentioned issues have to be handled for developing and maintaining any secure big data system that also considers privacy as one of its main concerns.

8.3   Challenges

As perceived, healthcare applications not only generate big data, but are also fraught with challenges. The challenges are daunting, but application developers have to be aware of the challenges so that they also propose ways of mitigating the challenge. A few challenges are identified here.

8.3.1   Malicious User

A user is usually validated when he logs into the system. Based on the access control policy, he is granted corresponding permissions. The suspicion that can never occur in the mind of the system administrator is that the user may do some wrong-doing in the system.

It may be really hard to believe that a user can have intentions of harming the system he is working on. But real-life experience tells us that a user may really become malicious during his lifetime. It is obvious that finding a valid user who actually does not have good intentions is pretty hard. However, steps must be taken to monitor the activities of each user and record any out-of-the-box activity of any user. The sessions when a user is active must be logged properly. Viewing logs and analysis of logs may identify an activity that does not follow the regular pattern of activities that this user performs. Then only that user may be singled out and appropriate measures may be taken against him. At first warnings may be issued and then he may be barred from system activities.

In a healthcare system, users are involved in different roles. Thus, there are several categories of users. Hence, even if any one user from any category turns out to be malicious, it would be detrimental to the system.

8.3.2 Identifying Threats

Mobile devices are ubiquitous and are widely used by all and sundry, from doctors, nurses, administrators, and caregiver staff, to patients and visitors. It is nevertheless essential to provide network access anywhere and anytime to ensure quality patient care. But this is also one of the most vulnerable points in the entire IT-based healthcare system. There are various threat sources to such applications. The responsibility of the healthcare industry lies in taking precautions against these threats. Hence, proper identification and verification of users as well as their devices becomes necessary.

Medical equipment such as medication scanners, patient-monitoring systems, and imaging devices are becoming more and more common. Each has embedded connectivity, thereby making the activities of tracking, monitoring, and managing enterprise productivity easier. These systems also help in reducing errors. Not only is embedded connectivity a burden on bandwidth, it also exposes the network to malware and viruses. This gives rise to new threats in the system. A large number of enterprises nowadays have a 'virtualisation' strategy that runs more than one application on one server. This is also true for healthcare enterprises. However, threats in such systems are the same as in any other networked system. Hence, the same sort of precautions should be taken.

8.3.3 Risk Mitigation

A number of risks are associated with any system. To identify each risk and plan for handling each risk is in itself a time-consuming task. Some risks may be identified in the design stage, and appropriate mitigation plans may be adopted accordingly. But some other risks may unfold with time. Managing these dynamic risks is definitely problematic.

Categories of risks may be identified and analysed in the design and planning stage. Stakeholders may be asked to identify all probable risks. The developers usually integrate the mitigation plans inside the system, so that no extra effort has to be taken in run-time. However, when risk occurs dynamically and all of a sudden, immediate and previously unplanned measures have to be taken. Hence the measures may or may not be able to contain the risk in totality. But the probability of this sudden occurrence of a till-now unidentified risk is very low, given all the other risks that have been pre-identified.

Hence, near-complete identification of risks during design and planning is of the utmost importance.

A few mitigation techniques are mentioned here. This is obviously not a complete set, and it is also not possible to build a complete risk mitigation set. The practice of *least privilege access*, that is, when users are given only those privileges they need to perform their jobs, is one such risk mitigation strategy. Organisations may also follow the principle of *need to know*. This means that no extra information other than the information actually needed will be provided. Another important strategy may be *auditing*. Equally important is supervising business partners so that they adhere to the security policies of the organisation.

8.3.4   Real-Time Monitoring

Most of the security incidents happen when the system is running. Hence real-time monitoring of the system is a necessity. Of course, it is very easy to describe but very difficult to implement. Real-time monitoring requires proper logging of (i) all incidents or events in the system, (ii) user activities, (iii) networking activities (network traffic), (iv) resource access, (v) requests for different activities, and so on. However, the complementary activity of real-time monitoring is taking appropriate action after identifying activity which does not fall under the category of routine activity. This sounds difficult, and it really is, because identifying an unusual activity and taking steps, all of these in real-time, is hard to implement.

8.3.5   Privacy Preservation

As mentioned in 8.1.2, *privacy* is one of the major concerns in healthcare applications.

Healthcare data encompasses different types of patient data for example from general information like name, address, age, height, and weight, to clinical test reports including graphical reports and/or images (ECG and USG) to diagnosis, and finally, to prescription. A patient may not want to reveal his medical condition for a number of reasons. The medical condition may be simple or sometimes fatal. Whatever the reasons, a person has every right not to disclose information to those who may not require it. This implies that his doctor and caregiver may know about his condition, but not any other person. We have to respect the patient's *privacy* in such situations.

At some other times, there may be binding agreements with the government not to disclose some medical information. In such cases, the relationship between the medical condition and the person with the medical condition is important. The aim of the government is to protect the person suffering from that medical condition, possibly from social stigma! At other times, research agencies or pharmaceutical companies may be interested to know about a disease prevalent in an area. They will not be interested to know about the names of the persons suffering from that disease. In such cases also, the names of the patients must not be revealed. This is also for protecting *privacy* of that patient.

There are several ways to protect the privacy of a data field. The simplest way of concealing data, and probably, individual data fields from others is *encryption*. Data fields may be encrypted using an encryption technique, and only the valid recipient will be able to read the data using the appropriate key. However, as discussed in 8.1.2 and above, it is interesting to note that association among the different fields may be of interest to the outside world. Since this seems inappropriate, measures have to be taken to guard the association.

One of the methods that may be used here is the creation of *metadata*. This data about actual data is not supposed to reveal the actual data. However, this means that the *metadata* itself has to be designed in such a way that it is a sort of wrapper over the actual data, and the outside world is aware of the wrapper only. Hence, any query will be on the *metadata*, which has to be transformed appropriately at some level for accessing the actual data.

Another interesting measure could be to encrypt all data fields and query such that data access will be on encrypted data. The result of the query will be encrypted data itself, to be decrypted by the proper recipient.

One of the widely used techniques for privacy preservation is *Homomorphic encryption* . Interestingly, this scheme encrypts data into ciphertext that can be analysed and even computed without the need for decrypting the data, and, also without even needing the decryption key. Further, mathematical operations can also be carried out on the ciphertext without compromising the encryption. The initial idea of *homomorphic encryption* was proposed by Rivest et al. [32]. Gentry [12] was the first to report Fully Homomorphic Encryption (FHE) scheme that was capable of performing multiplications and additions.

However, still other techniques [1] are there for privacy preservation. The work in [37] discusses *anonymisation* and *encryption* methods for privacy preservation of healthcare data.

The U.S. Government has already enacted the *Health Insurance Portability and Accountability Act* (HIPAA) [20] which took effect in April 2003. This law is designed to provide privacy standards to protect patients' medical records and other health information provided to health plans, doctors, hospitals, and other health care providers. These new standards not only provide patients with access to their medical records, but also allow them to exercise more control over how their personal health information can be used and disclosed.

8.3.5.1   Health Data Sale

It is really frightening to see how data breaches occur and to whom this data goes. This can indicate how the data is used. For example, stolen data may be used to generate fraudulent healthcare bills and prescriptions, and credit card transactions for purchasing items, to modify health records, and so on [15].

The healthcare industry faces challenges due to the presence of ruthless hackers. Patient Health Information (PHI) includes all the relevant information about an individual. Hence, although patient safety may not be directly related to data security this is actually the case, given the amount of information PHI contains. The reports of data breaches circulating in the media a couple of years back were very disturbing. The healthcare industry has experienced a number of breaches in the past few years. The price of stolen health data is much more than the price of stolen credit card numbers on the black market. The reason may lie in the fact that a stolen credit card will be cancelled and other steps taken in due time. But for stolen health information, what can the victim do to protect himself?

The stolen health data records are used for identity theft, for (i) credentials, (ii) a complete electronic dossier, (iii) a custom-made fraudulent kit from (ii). But it must be noted that hacking is not the only means of compromising medical information. Healthcare workers may steal data, or worse; relatives or friends may also use information to obtain fake medical claims. Health insurance information, on the other hand, may be used to purchase medical equipment and drugs, to be sold again illegally.

Regardless of the industries involved, identity theft is always a big scare.

Generally, healthcare organisation insiders have a knowledge about the sophistication of the attacks, and hence, adopt even fewer security measures. So it is only natural and no surprise to guess, that they are targeted and compromised much more easily. Vulnerabilities are visible everywhere with the use of common tools, network, frameworks, data storage, and sharing. People also have the idea that only financial data is valuable, and hence, needs to be protected. So, less attention is given to other data in an organisation. Hence, data may not be encrypted at all and may be stored in the open. Even HIPAA does not provide any mandate about encrypting data, though it looks after patient privacy issues.

8.3.5.2   Compliance for EHR

A regulatory compliance program is necessary to control security-related malpractice in healthcare organisations [15]. However, management or some central authorities have to coordinate such programs. The tasks are numerous, from gathering information about controls used and testing, to developing a set of objectives to be followed by all, and coordination of the overall activities. Only some mature organisations realise that they have to look into the matter from the perspective of risk and focus more on areas with higher risks. In the United States, the revised HIPAA now requires providers to assess the security of their databases, applications, and systems containing patient information. It has also mentioned a list of 75 specific controls as safeguards. But what about other nations with no such law in practice?

8.4 Security of NoSQL Databases

A large number of companies are adopting big data solutions now. However, they have concerns regarding what to use – Hadoop or Spark, NoSQL database or the RDBMS they are currently using. Everyone is still not convinced to follow the current technology trend. NoSQL databases are designed to store and process large amounts of unstructured data, a requirement for many current applications. It is highly scalable, with high availability. There may be many other factors influencing the choice of NoSQL over RDBMS for current scenarios.

8.4.1 Reviewing Security in NoSQL databases

Eric Brewer [6] introduced the CAP theorem, which mentions three properties of shared-data systems, namely data consistency, system availability, and tolerance to network partitions. Traditional DBMS designers always prioritized the properties of consistency and availability. But now, with changes in the perspective of data storage, it seems that focusing on the network aspects is necessary. Hence, tolerance to network partitions has to be the focus.

Here we first focus on Cassandra [18] and MongoDB [23], each with its own distinctive features. We also discuss HBase [40], which is built on top of the Hadoop File System (HDFS).

Cassandra is known for managing huge amounts of structured data spread across commodity servers. It is a distributed storage system providing highly available service. Cassandra does not have single point of failure. Although its components may often fail, Cassandra is designed in such a way that it survives failures. MongoDB is a document database. It manages collections of JSON-like documents. Documents are stored in collections, and collections in turn are stored in a database. Although collection is similar to table in

RDBMS, MongoDB lacks any schema. Shardings and Replica sets are used by MongoDB that provide high availability and scalability.

Cassandra and MongoDB are now widely used for research-oriented activities as well as enterprise solutions. All these activities tend to store large amounts of user-related sensitive information. This raises concerns regarding confidentiality and privacy of the data and the security provided by these systems.

The main problems as detailed below and faced by both systems include lack of encryption support for the data files, weak authentication, simple authorisation without support for RBAC or fine-grained authorisation, and vulnerability to injection and Denial of Service (DoS) attacks.

8.4.1.1 Security in Cassandra

A review [11] of Cassandra security features revealed security vulnerabilities on the components mentioned below.

1. Data in Cassandra is kept unencrypted. So, anybody with filesystem access can access data, and if he is a malicious user, then data may be used for unethical purposes.

2. In general, unencrypted communication is the norm between the database and its client. Monitoring database traffic is not a difficult task and hence data may be viewed by an attacker as well.

3. In general, nodes on a cluster communicate without using any encryption or authentication. Also, no protection or authentication is provided to the interface that is used to load bulk data into Cassandra from different nodes in the cluster.

4. Cassandra Query Language (CQL) API should be checked, since it may be vulnerable to injection attack.

5. An attacker may take up all the resources of a server in fake connection requests, thereby compelling the server to refuse new connections. This ultimately leads to the Denial of Service i.e, DoS attack.

6. It is possible for an attacker that can sniff out communication between a legitimate client and the database to be able to retrieve passwords.

7. Generally, authorisation in Cassandra is specified only on existing column families. There is no mention about protection on newly added column families and columns.

8. Inline auditing is also not provided in Cassandra.

Cassandra now provides security features [9] [36] as mentioned below, to handle the above-mentioned issues.

1. Authentication provided by Cassandra is role-based and stored internally in Cassandra system tables.

2. Role authentication has become the crux. Authorisation for access privileges are based on role authentication. Authorisation can be to access the entire database or restrict a role to individual table access. Roles can grant authorisation to authorise other roles.

3. Cassandra now provides secure communication between client and database cluster, and between nodes in a cluster. TLS or SSL encryption is used to ensure that data in transit is not compromised. Client-to-node and node-to-node encryption are independently configured.

The authors in [21] described Security As Service and offered (i) Fine-grained column level authorisation, (ii) Encryption of data at rest, and (iii) Secure communication between entities. Cassandra is being used as the case study in this work. The authors identified the threats that can be protected. They also analysed the working of the protocol under a couple of attacks.

8.4.1.2 Security in MongoDB

The authors in [11] analysed the security features of MongoDB. The security vulnerabilities on the undermentioned components were noted by them. The authors also suggested some mitigation techniques or plans to do away with the threats.

1. Data files in MongoDB are not kept encrypted. So, any user with file-system access is able to get hold of data. He can misuse data if he does not have good intentions. Therefore, the application must explicitly encrypt any sensitive information before saving it. Also, operating-system access control mechanisms are to be used to prevent unauthorised access.

2. MongoDB uses a TCP port by default, which is used by the wire-level protocol it supports. This protocol is neither encrypted nor compressed. The internal HTTP server also doesn't support TLS or SSL. However, an HTTP proxy server like Apache HTTPD can be used instead. This would enable use of the Apache HTTPD's authentication and authorisation support, in addition to robust SSL encryption for the connection.

3. MongoDB uses JavaScript as the internal scripting language. Because JavaScript is an interpreted language, there is a probability of injection attacks.

4. MongoDB doesn't support authentication in *sharded* mode. But in standalone or replica-set mode, authentication can be enabled in MongoDB. In replica-set mode, not only the clients authenticate to the database, but each replica server also has to authenticate to the

other servers before joining the cluster. In both modes, authentication is based on a pre-shared secret. The way in which passwords are stored paves the way for an attacker to easily recover the entire set. The use of a proxy server may be helpful here.

5. In Sharded mode, MongoDB doesn't support authentication, and therefore has no support for authorisation. Authentication, Authorisation, and Auditing are possible if configured on reverse proxy.

6. MongoDB doesnt provide any facilities for auditing actions performed in the database. MongoDB just puts a one-liner in the log for a new namespace, but nothing more subsequently.

8.4.1.3 Security in HBase

Apache HBase is used for random, real-time read or write access to big data. HBase is internally used by many companies, such as Facebook, Twitter, Yahoo, and Adobe. Users can be granted permission, and permission can be revoked as well.

Below is a list of the privileges that can be provided to a user in HBase. Access levels are granted independently of each other and allow for different types of operations at a given scope [8].

1. R: Read privilege

2. W: Write privilege

3. X: Execute privilege

4. C: Create privilege

5. A: Admin privilege

The possible scopes as provided in HBase are:

1. Superuser – A *superuser* is able to perform any operation on any resource.

2. Global – Admin (the Administrator) is allowed to operate on all tables of the cluster if permissions is granted at *global* scope.

3. Namespace – Permissions granted at *namespace* scope apply to all tables within the given namespace.

4. Table – *Table*-scope-based permissions are applicable to data or metadata within a given table.

5. ColumnFamily – Permissions granted in *ColumnFamily* scope apply to cells within the particular ColumnFamily.

6. Cell – The *cell* scope permissions are applicable to exactly that particular cell coordinate. This allows for policy evolution along with data.

Possible access levels that can be granted to a user are created by the combination of access levels and scopes (as if in a matrix form). Access levels may basically denote what is needed to do a particular specific task. The *need to know* policy may be used, and more access than is required for a given user to perform their required tasks is not granted. Access levels for some categories of HBase users is as follows:

1. Superusers – An HBase user should only have superuser access. However, during development, an administrator may need superuser access such that he can control and manage the cluster. But this type of access for the administrator may be done as *global admin*.

2. Global Admins – A global admin is allowed to perform tasks and access every table in HBase. Typically, an admin would not have Read or Write permissions for data in the tables. However, global admin with *Admin* permissions can perform cluster-wide operations on the cluster. These operations include balancing, assigning, or removing regions, or calling an explicit major compaction. This is an operations type of role. A global admin with *Create* permissions can create or drop any table within HBase. This is something like the role of a Database Administrator.

3. Table Admins – As the role suggests, a table admin has access to and can perform administrative operations only on that particular table. A table admin may have different permissions; Create permissions can be used to create snapshots from that table or restore that table from a snapshot. Similarly, with *Admin* permissions, a table admin can perform operations like splits or major compactions on that table.

4. Users – Users can read or write data, or both. Users can also be given Executable permissions, and are able to execute coprocessor endpoints.

Default HBase [3] configuration allows every user to read from and write to all tables. Obviously, this is not desirable. Although setting up *firewalls* may partially address the problems, it is not effective enough because HBase still is unable to differentiate between multiple users that use the same client machines, and there is no granularity regarding HBase table, column family, or column qualifier access.

User *authentication* can be implemented whereby *authorised* users are only allowed to communicate with HBase. The authorisation system at Remote Procedure Call level, is based on the Simple Authentication and Security Layer (SASL). Kerberos [22] is supported in SASL, which allows authentication, encryption negotiation, and message integrity verification. These are based per connection. User *authentication* is completed here. The Admin then gets the ability to define a series of User *authorisation* rules that allow or deny individual actions. The Authorisation system is also known as the *Access Controller Coprocessor* or *Access Control List* (ACL). It gives the ability to define authorisation policy with granularity, for a specified user.

As an example, it can be said that (i) an administrator in *Global* scope with *Create* permissions is able to do the following: create tables and provide access to Table Administrators; or, (ii) a data analyst in *Table* scope with *Read* permissions can perform the following: read HBase and create reports from HBase data.

8.4.2   Reviewing Enterprise Approaches towards Security in NoSQL Databases

Security has always been a major concern for IT enterprises, regardless of the application domains. A number of security issues [26] associated with NoSQL databases have come up. These issues span across different NoSQL databases. The list mentioned below is not at all exhaustive. Many issues are coming up with each new day:

1. Weak authentication between server and client

2. Weak password storage

3. Plaintext communication between client and server

4. Lack of encryption support

5. Unencrypted data at rest

6. External security cannot always be used

7. Vulnerable to DoS attack

It is apparent that although NoSQL databases are on the way to popularity, they are still new and may require much polishing to be presented as a finished product! NoSQL databases are in the evolutionary stage, and hence, attack vectors may still not be mapped out. There are chances of new attack vectors targeting NoSQL coming up in the future. However, it is always necessary and advisable to evaluate security and other related application requirements before choosing any database! It also seems that NoSQL is not more or less secure than RDBMS.

Different enterprises that provide NoSQL databases, tools, and support, also try to pack some security solutions [26]. These may include the following; however, this list is ever growing.

1. Include security policies

2. Define Users and Groups

3. Grant permission only after authentication

4. Secure communication (using encryption) from client machine to database cluster

5. Client-to-server SSL

6. An external security tool like Kerberos [22] may be configured and used

7. Transparent data encryption for data at rest

Mitigating security risks [33] in NoSQL systems is always important. A secure software may include the above-mentioned security solutions. It also helps if the developer is aware of the weaknesses in the system, because then he will try to improve upon that. This also needs the requirements of protections and a clear idea about what needs to be protected. The development must use the best practices of writing safe code by using well-validated shared libraries and libraries for encryption.

As of now, there may not be any standardised authentication practice for NoSQL databases. The approach in such situations can be to view security as a middleware layer. This will be helpful, as most middleware software comes with support for authentication, authorisation, and access control [41]. However, managing proper authentication and role-based access control authorisation on popular NoSQL databases is now coming up. Dynamic and static application security testing (DAST and SAST, respectively) may also be executed on the application or source code to find injection vulnerabilities. An important but overlooked part of protecting the application is ensuring a secure deployment.

8.5 Integrating Security with Big Data Solutions

Much has been said about the requirements of security in big data system solution. This section at first summarizes the *why* and *how* of big data security solutions.

It is expected that big data breaches may have far-reaching and devastating effects because of their nature. It may be that breaches will affect larger sections of people, and hence, may create legal challenges, too. For privacy purposes, if the data is anonymised, it must adhere to required quality. Also, data may not be stored in the *open* and may have to be *encrypted*. The requirement may be to perform operations on encrypted data without having any knowledge about the underlying data. The data owners and the data storage owners may face challenges regarding ownership and providing requirements of security. It is to be made clear that both parties should have responsibility; while data owners may put restrictions on data access, storage providers may try to secure data at rest.

Big data solutions often rely on firewalls or implementations at the application layer to provide or restrict access to information. Although access control has traditionally been provided by operating systems, designers on behalf of the applications can also restrict the way data will be accessed. An easy and simple approach may be to use encryption on data that can only be decrypted by an *authorised* entity. Of course, *authorisation* will be provided through the access control policy. *Attribute-based Encryption* (ABE) is another method that takes data or user attributes into account and encrypts accordingly. ABE may be applied once sensitive data attributes are identified.

A big data system may have numerous different types of users, each requiring some particular information or subset of information. This implies that access control needs to be granular to incorporate these new conditions.

Real-time security monitoring is also important for any big data system. But without threat intelligence, this monitoring may not be effective, since attacks may not be detected in time for the system to react appropriately [17].

8.5.1   Big Data Enterprise Security

Now the time has come to look at security from the perspective of enterprise. The big data platform used for storing big data also stores all the insights, patterns, and analytics results that have been derived or discovered from this big data [19]. So, what is Enterprise security? Enterprise security is mainly concerned with security to data or information and the entities related to that. So, it encompasses the entities in which data is generated or stored, or the path the data travels. The storage may be cloud storage, too.

The key verticals [19] of enterprise security include: *Infrastructure security, Network security, System security, Authentication, Authorization, Access control, Encryption and masking, Audit and monitoring*. Any big data solution in an enterprise will have to address these verticals. Only then it can be said that it is a *secure* big data enterprise solution.

Enterprise security is driven by three things [19]: *Legislation, Internal policies*, and *Business drivers*. The *Legislation* requirement is for forcing some regulatory and standard compliance on the enterprises. Without it, the enterprises may behave according to their own rules. The regulations and compliance may follow global laws or local laws, whichever is appropriate. A few of the global standards are mentioned below:

1. ISO/IEC 27002:2005: Code of Practice for Information Security Management

2. HIPAA: Health Insurance Portability and Accountability Act 1996 (USA) (mentioned in 8.3.5)

3. Data Protection Act of 1984, amended 1998 (UK)

4. Data Protection Act of 1978, revised in 2004 (France)

5. Federal Data Protection Act (Bundesdatenschutzgesetz BDSG) 2017 (Germany)

6. European General Data Protection Regulation (GDPR: approved by the EU Parliament on April 14, 2016; Enforcement date: May 25, 2018)

ISO/IEC 27002:2005 [16] is published by ISO (International Organisation for Standardisation) and IEC (International Electrotechnical Commission). The title is: Information technology Security techniques Code of practice for information security controls. This provides best practice recommendations on information security controls for use in information security management systems.

The Data Protection Act of 1984, amended 1998 (UK) [27] is designed to protect personal data stored in various media. It follows the EU Data Protection Directive of 1995.

The French Data Protection Act of 1978 (revised 2004) [31] focuses on the principles of quality of personal data, legitimacy of data processing, stronger protection for special categories of data, obligation of information and rights of data subjects, security obligations for processing, data protection authorities, and data exchanges with countries outside the EU.

The new Federal Data Protection Act (Bundesdatenschutzgesetz BDSG) [42], released on April 27, 2017, consists of the following parts:

1. joint provisions,

2. implementing provisions for the GDPR,

3. transposition of the Directive for data protection for the purposes of prevention, and prosecution of criminal offences, and

4. special provisions for processing, which is not subject to the European regulations.

The General Data Protection Regulation [29] (GDPR) (EU) 2016/679 is a regulation in European Union (EU) law. This regulation is regarding data protection and privacy for all individuals within the EU and export of personal data outside the EU. The aim of the GDPR is to primarily provide control to citizens and residents over their personal data.

It is always to be remembered that most security technologies are not foolproof. Traditional IT security does not always have a defined structured approach and focuses on network security only, rather than having a holistic approach.

The white paper [28] describes a comprehensive big data security strategy from Oracle and Intel that focuses on *controls*, with an aim towards protecting big data environments at multiple levels.

1. Preventive Control: *Preventive* controls are somewhat proactive in nature. These are predesigned to prohibit unauthorised activities.

2. Detective Control: *Detective* control is the mechanism used to find problems in the system or the processes of the system and report them accordingly.

3. Administrative Control: *Administrative* controls are meant to have a clear picture of all the components of the system, and in particular, the protection of sensitive data and its storage.

An important *control* is the *Corrective* control. It may be used to act in conjunction with the Preventive and Detective controls. Corrective controls provide the mitigation for damage when breaches do occur.

The Oracle-Intel solution uses in-memory processing for big data analytics and chip-layer encryption. The combination of these layered, defense-in-depth solutions from both analytics and encryption, ensures data privacy and protection against insider threats.

The Hadoop ecosystem has Knox and Ranger as its two important security supports [5]. Knox provides a security management framework and supports security implementations, such as authorisation management, monitoring, and auditing, on Hadoop clusters. The Ranger provides a centralised framework that can be used to manage policies regarding resources. Ranger helps administrators implement access policies. It has different authorisation functionality for different Hadoop components, such as YARN, HBase, Hive, etc.

Current versions of Hadoop provide end-to-end encryption for data at rest within the Hadoop cluster and also in motion across the network. Hadoop supports encryption at different levels: disk, file system, database, and application levels.

8.6   Secured Health Data Delivery: A Case Study

This section considers remote health care applications for patients in villages in India. It describes the approach towards overall security of the application. In this remote health care application, patient health data is collected at remote locations using either body area network (BAN, as described in Chapter 3) or health kits provided by healthcare personnel. The health kit may contain several different types of sensor-based equipment to note several physiological parameters. First, basic information of the patient, like name, age, address, height, weight, and previous history of illness (if any) are noted. Other parameters are measured through the health kit and symptoms noted down accordingly. This patient health information is uploaded to cloud storage in a timely manner, so that it is available to appropriate authorised users including doctors, as and when necessary. A Cloud Service Provider (CSP) will provide the required cloud services, including cloud storage, to be provided by a Storage Provider (SP). Often, these health records contain sensitive data in terms of social, ethical, and legal aspects of medical science. Hence, it must be mandatory to keep this data protected from unauthorised access and disclosure. There are various stages this data passes through. The privacy of the patient data must therefore be maintained during data transmission, data storage, and data access. Hence, care has to be taken for data during transmission (channels and network), for data at rest (storage servers) and for data access (via query) as well.

Since we may assume that channels are not safe, a safeguard has to be added during transmission to provide confidentiality. The issue of integrity must also be taken care of during transmission. The data may be encrypted and then stored. Data access must be designed in such a manner that only authorised personnel is able to access the data. The doctor or health care personnel should be able to access the patient data stored in the cloud storage and generate the medical health reports and advice accordingly. Based on this analysis, the treatment is carried out.

The challenge is to maintain all security parameters and control the overhead while providing fast and timely access. The work in [34] and [25] describes a framework for data confidentiality and fine grained access methodology for a cloud-based remote health care application.

The task of the Cloud Service Provider (CSP) involves also more than one phase. The tasks will be to: 1. Collect credentials of new users and store the credentials for each user in secured storage, and secondly: 2. Authenticate the remote user before giving him or her access to the network, and thereby storage. Apart from the CSP, there is also a role for the Storage Provider

(SP). The CSP is considered to be different from the SP, in the sense that the CSP will have services other than storage to provide. However, it becomes important that both the CSP and the SP should *know* each other. This implies that whenever an SP registers itself with the CSP, they exchange suitable information based on which symmetric keys will be generated. This may be accomplished during initial handshaking.

The protocol described below will be used for different registration and authentication purposes, such as CSP-SP registration, CSP-user registration, and user authentication. Hence, it will be executed in different phases. As described above, the first phase deals with the CSP and the SPs.

Phase I: Each SP registers with the CSP. (It is to be noted here that there are several SPs). Handshaking information between the SP and CSP will be used for generating a symmetric key.

Phase II: New User registration (with CSP): It is assumed that the new user will be allocated a proper SP whenever he registers.

1. Generation of credentials of user by CSP
2. CSP encrypts information
3. CSP sends it to SP (for later use)
4. SP stores encrypted information

Phase I and Phase II will be executed only once during new SP registration with CSP, and during new user registration with CSP, respectively.

Phase III: User request to CSP (query regarding data):

1. CSP asks SP for user information
2. SP retrieves encrypted information from its storage
3. SP sends encrypted information to CSP
4. CSP authenticates user

Phase IV: User is granted request provided authentication is successful.

During phase I when SP_k registers with the CSP, symmetric key $S1_k$ is generated. In phase II, user information (registration details) are encrypted with $S1_k$ by CSP and stored with SP_k. Similarly, in phase III, when the user requests data access, he has to be authenticated first. SP_k retrieves encrypted user information and sends it to the CSP. the CSP compares the saved information with the newly entered information. CSP authenticates the user when these match.

Health information of an individual (patient) may contain some sensitive data which must not be accessed by all users. Therefore, some restrictions should be in place to control data access. A simple methodology is described here.

The data is first segmented into parts based on the sensitivity of the information. Each data segment contains some specific information about the patient's health. Whenever a user requests information, the entire health information may not be shown or made accessible to him. He requires permission to access the part or the entire data. Permission is given based on the user role, data sensitivity, and data access policy. Thus, restricted access to data is achieved.

We assume here that the first segment of patient data contains header information. Another part contains a detailed description about the patient and his health-related information. The second part is again partitioned into a couple of segments (based on sensitivity) for better access management strategy. This implies that a user will receive an appropriate key for accessing the data he is authorised to access.

The work in [34] describes the secure flow of data in the remote healthcare application. To achieve this secure flow, a double layered technique is used. The data is assumed to be segmented into three parts (Segment1, Segment2, Segment3, and a Header). AES [13] is used for encrypting different segments of patient data using different symmetric keys (each 128 bit), K_{SEG1}, K_{SEG2}, K_{SEG3}. Since this is a symmetric key encryption, users will also need these keys. But the keys will not be provided to all and sundry. These are provided to authorised users only, and that too on an on-demand basis.

Another layer of AES is applied to the data before transmission. This time the key is derived at both ends during run time. An asymmetric key technique is used in this stage to generate the new symmetric key. The symmetric key distribution is done in an asymmetric fashion. One public and one private key pair is generated each time before transmission. Using these values, at each end, one ephemeral shared secret is generated, which is used to derive the symmetric key. This key is further used to encrypt the patient record. This asymmetric key generation technique also helps in signing the data using the generated private part.

After successful user authentication that may also include verification of his role in the system, authorisation will be provided to the user. This includes providing the user with the proper access key, so that the user could retrieve the data he has access to. As mentioned above, when the data [Header +

Segment1 + Segment2 + Segment3] is sent to the cloud storage, a run time symmetric key is generated (at both ends), which is used to encrypt the data at the sender side. On the other side, the cloud storage provider can decrypt the data. The decrypted data is actually segmented encrypted data with a header. The storage provider (SP) creates one metadata information using the received header. Then, again it encrypts the data with its symmetric storage key and stores the data.

At the time of access, the user sends a query about patient data to the storage provider (SP) via the cloud service provider (CSP). The CSP sends the query in encrypted form (using their symmetric key) to the SP. The SP decrypts the query, checks user authorisation, and searches the metadata information. Upon retrieval of the requested patient data, the decrypted data (decryption using the storage key) is further encrypted using the user's symmetric key. The encrypted data is now sent back from the SP to the user via the CSP. Users are provided with these access keys on demand. The data can now be decrypted only by the intended user. However, provision is also present to grant proper permission (read, write) on the data based on the user's role. Therefore, the intended data is visible (as per permission granted) only at the user's end.

The work in [34] also mentions the different messages that are exchanged in the secure framework for remote healthcare application. This framework provides confidentiality to data and controls access to users. It first guarantees that actual data is not available to unauthorised users and then guarantees that without proper permission, operations on data will not be allowed. Hence, none other than the doctor D assigned to patient P is able to write or modify the prescription. The patient P will be able to read the prescription only.

It is quite apparent that data retrieval from cloud storage (representing a shared resources environment) by different users may blend data from different requests in a single place. Here lies the need for an efficient and secure data retrieval strategy by different users (probably at the same time). When sensitive information is transmitted over the network, there is high probability of information leakage.

For simultaneous data access by multiple users, the requirement is that each user request be handled in a logically separate fashion [35]. Therefore, while executing user requests, it must be ensured that the same task for different users, such as user validation module for task A and user validation module for task B, must be executed separately, so that the output of task A or task B cannot be inferred by any other (curious!) task.

A glimpse of secured health data delivery is described in this section. It provides an overview of the entire scenario by considering data storage in the cloud to be accessed by different categories of users for uploading health data, including text and images, modifying data depending upon current symptoms and pathological results, writing prescriptions by accessing the stored data, and so on.

8.7 Chapter Notes

Security of health data is one of the main concerns. This chapter deals in details of how health data can be securely stored and accessed by various types of users. Since users are different and have varying requirements, access permission also depends upon a number of parameters, from the role of the user to data attributes. The chapter finally describes a security framework for remote healthcare application that is able to deliver secured health data. Privacy preservation and data confidentiality, along with handling of simultaneous access requests, here with are dealt.

However, there still remains a plethora of other related (directly or indirectly) issues that need attention in order to develop a secure, fool-proof, privacy-preserving healthcare data delivery system.

References

[1] N. Adam, T. White, and et al. Privacy Preserving Integration of Health Care Data. In *AMIA Annual Symposium Proceedings*, pages 1–5, 2007.

[2] Elisa Bertino, Ji-Won Byun, and Ninghui Li. Privacy-preserving database systems. *FOS AD*, pages 178–206, 2005.

[3] Matteo Bertozzi. How-to: Enable user authentication and authorization in apache hbase. Website: http://blog.cloudera.com/blog/2012/09/understanding-user-authentication-and-authorization-in-apache-hbase/, 2012.

[4] Matt Bishop. *Computer Security: Art and Science*. Addison Wesley, 2002.

[5] BMCSoftware. Introduction to Hadoop Security. Website: http://www.bmcsoftware.in/guides/hadoop-security.html, 2016.

[6] Eric Brewer. Towards robust distributed system. Website: https://dl.acm.org/citation.cfm?id=343502, 2000.

[7] C. Clifton and J. Vaidya. Privacy-preserving data mining: Why, how, and when. *IEEE Security and Privacy*, 2(6):19–27, 2004.

[8] Cloudera. Managing HBase Security. Website: https://www.cloudera.com/documentation/enterprise/5-6-x/topics/security.html, 2017.

[9] Datastax. Securing Cassandra. Website: https://docs.datastax.com/en/cassandra/3.0/cassandra/configuration/secureIntro.html, 2018.

[10] Kevvie Fowler. Big Data Security. Website: http://docplayer.net/2780740-Big-data-security-kevvie-fowler-kpmg-ca.html, 2013.

[11] Nurit Gal-Oz and Yaron Gonen. Security Issues in NoSQL Databases. In *2011 International Joint Conference of IEEE TrustCom-11 IEEE ICESS-11-FCST-11*, pages 541–547, 2011.

[12] C. Gentry. Fully homomorphic encryption using ideal lattices. In *41st Annual ACM Symposium on Theory of Computing*, pages 169–178, 2009.

[13] R. Housley. Advanced Encryption Standard (AES) Key Wrap Algorithm. *No. RFC 3394*, 2002.

[14] IBM. Authentication. Website: `https://www.ibm.com/support/knowledgecenter/en/SS6RHZ\_1.1.2/com.ibm.rational.pe.administer.doc/topics/c\_authentication.html`, 2016.

[15] InfoSecInstitute. Incident response. Website: `http://resources.infosecinstitute.com/hackers-selling-healthcare-data-in-the-black-market/\#gref`, 2015.

[16] ISO/IEC JTC1/SC27. ISO/IEC 27002. Website: `https://en.wikipedia.org/wiki/ISO/IEC\_27002`, 2013.

[17] Guillermo Lafuente. Big Data Security – Challenges & Solutions. Website: `https://www.mwrinfosecurity.com/our-thinking/big-data-security-challenges-and-solutions/`, November 2014.

[18] A. Lakshman and P. Malik. Cassandra: a decentralized structured storage system. *SIGOPS Operating Systems Review*, 7(4):35–40, 2010.

[19] Andrew Lion. Big data-biggest risk. Website: `https://www.hadoop360.datasciencecentral.com/blog/big-data-biggest-security-risk`, 2014.

[20] MedTerms. Medical Dictionary. Website: `https://www.medicinenet.com/script/main/art.asp?articlekey=31785`, 2016.

[21] F. Mehak, R. Masood, and et al. Security Aspects of Database-as-a-Service (DBaaS) in Cloud Computing. In Z. Mahmood, editor, *Cloud Computing*. Computer Communications and Networks, 2014.

[22] MIT. Kerberos: The network authentication protocol. Website: `http://web.mit.edu/kerberos/`, 2017.

[23] mongoDB. mongoDB : for Giant Ideas. Website: `http://www.mongodb.org/`, 2016.

[24] Sam Narisi. 10 best practices to secure healthcare data. Website: `http://www.healthcarebusinesstech.com/best-practices-to-secure-healthcare-data/`, 2013.

[25] Sarmistha Neogy and Sayantani Saha. Developing a secure remote patient monitoring system. In *IEEE Xplore International Conference on Cyber Security and Protection of Digital Services (Cyber Security 2015)*, pages 1–4, 2015.

[26] Mike Obijaju. Nosql no security - security issues with nosql database. Website: `http://blogs.perficient.com`, 2015.

[27] Parliament of the United Kingdom. Data Protection Act 1998. Website: https://www.legislation.gov.uk/ukpga/1998/29/contents, 1998.

[28] Oracle and Intel. Enterprise Security for Big Data Environments: A Multi-Layered Approach for Defense-in-Depth Protection. Website: http://www.oracle.com/us/technologies/big-data/big-data-security-wp-3099503.pdf, July 2016.

[29] European Parliament and Council. General data protection regulation. Website: https://en.wikipedia.org/wiki/General_Data_Protection_Regulation, 2016.

[30] *R. Agrawal, J. Kiernan,* and et al. Hippocratic databases. In *28th International Conference on Very Large Databases (VLDB),* 2002.

[31] Pascale Rauline-Serrier. CNIL: The French Data Protection Authority. Website: https://www.americanbar.org/content/dam/aba/publications/antitrust_law/20130617_at13617_materials.authcheckdam.pdf, 2004.

[32] R. L. Rivest, L. Adleman, and M. L. Dertouzos. On data banks and Privacy Homomorphisms. *Foundations of Secure Computation,* 4(11):169–179, 1978.

[33] Aviv Ron, Alexandra-Shulman-Peleg, and Anton Puzanov. Analysis and Mitigation of NoSQL Injections. Website: https://www.infoq.com/articles/nosql-injections-analysis, January 2017.

[34] Sayantani Saha, Rounak Das, Suman Datta, and Sarmistha Neogy. A Cloud Security Framework for a Data centric WSN Application. In *ACM Digital Library Proceedings of the 17th International Conference on Distributed Computing and Networking.*

[35] Sayantani Saha, Tanusree Parbat, and Sarmistha Neogy. Designing a Secure Data Retrieval Strategy Using NoSQL Database. In Parida L. Krishnan P., Radha Krishna P., editor, *Distributed Computing and Internet Technology. ICDCIT 2017: Lecture Notes in Computer Science,* volume 10109. Springer, Cham, 2017.

[36] Security. Securing Cassandra. Website: http://cassandra.apache.org/doc/latest/operating/security.html, 2016.

[37] Bhanumati Selvaraj and Sakthivel Periyasamy. A Review of Recent Advances in Privacy Preservation in Healthcare Data Publishing. *International Journal of Pharma and Bio Sciences,* 7(4):33–41, 2016.

[38] L. Sweeney. Achieving k-anonymity privacy protection using generalization and suppression. *International Journal on Uncertainty, Fuzziness and Knowledge-based Systems,* 10(5):571–588, 2002.

[39] Symantech. Article-Support. Website: `https://support.symantec.com/en\_US/article.HOWTO92605{\#}v24644013.html`, 2013.

[40] Tutorialspoint. HBase Tutorial. Website: `https://www.tutorialspoint.com/hbase/hbase-overview.htm`, 2017.

[41] Davy Winder. Securing nosql applications: Best practices for big data security. Website: `http://computerweekly.com`, 2012.

[42] Tim Wybitul. Germany publishes English version of National GDPR Implementation Act. Website: `https://www.hldataprotection.com/articles/international-eu-privacy/`, 2017.

Index

access control, 203
ACID properties, 173
activation function, 93
Amdahl's law, 134
ANN in medical domain, 96
ANN mode, 92
ANN Model, 90
ANN structure, 93
ANN weakness, 97
anonymisation, 195
applications of big data, 55
Apriori algorithm, 112
ARM in health data, 113
ARM: issues, 114
ARM: performance, 114
ARMA, 117
Artificial Neural Network (ANN), 90
Association Rule Mining, 111
ASTM, 16
Attribute-based Access Control, 204
availability, 193

Back Propagation Neural Network, 93
Beowulf cluster, 139
Big Data, 8, 13, 43, 44, 54
big data processing, 130
big data security, 57, 59
big data solution, 185
Bluetooth, 70

Cassandra, 174, 185, 214
CEN, 16
cloud computing, 130
clustering, 98
column family, 185, 186
column-oriented databases, 174
communication cost, 133

composite key, 187
computation cost, 133
confidence, 112
confidentiality, 192
conviction, 112
cost, 131
CouchDB, 173
crowdsourcing, 76
CUDA architecture, 140

data model, 184
data parallelism, 143
data sensitivity, 200, 225
data structure stores, 168
decision tree, 106
demographic information, 23
denormalisation, 185
Discretionary Access Control (DAC), 204
distributed architecture, 136
document databases, 167, 168

efficiency, 132
eHealth, 2
eHealth solutions, 3
eHealthcare, 8
EHR, 14
EHR standards, 16, 30
EHR system, 15
EHR-S, 15
Electronic Health Record, 14
Electronic Medical Records, 15
EMR, 15
EN 13606, 17
EN13606 Archetypes, 17
EN13606 Reference Model, 17
entropy, 107

233

eventual consistency, 177

GINI index, 107
graph databases, 181
graph stores, 168

Hadoop, 179
Hadoop Distributed File System, 179
Hadoop YARN, 149
HBase, 179, 216
HDFS, 151, 179
health data, 13, 51, 166
health informatics, 5
health IT, 5
healthcare, 51, 52
healthcare crowdsourcing, 77
HIPAA, 211–213, 221
HL7, 16
HL7 CCD, 18
HL7 CDA, 18, 22
HL7 Clinical Document Architecture,
    18, 22
HL7 Continuity of Care Documents,
    18
HL7 messaging standards, 18, 19
HL7 reference information model, 20,
    21
homomorphic encryption, 211

ID3 algorithm, 108
IEEE 802.15.6, 71
integrity, 192
inverse document frequency, 122
ISO, 16
ISO 13606, 17
ISO TC-215 standards, 18
ISO/EN 13606, 18
itemset, 112

k-anonymity, 195
k-means clustering, 99
k-means clustering - remarks, 100
key-value databases, 167

Latent Dirichlet Allocation, 123
lift, 112

map function, 146
marginal linear model, 119
MEMS, 70
message passing model, 143
metadata, 211, 226
mobile health, 5
MongoDB, 169, 215
multicomputer, 136
multiprogramming model, 142

Naive Bayesian classification, 102
Naive Bayesian in medical data, 104
Neo4j, 181
non-uniform memory access, 137
NoSQL, 166
NoSQL databases, 167, 213
NUMA, 137

ontology, 32
openEHR archetypes, 26
openEHR reference information model,
    23
openEHR reference model, 26
openEHR templates, 28
OSI model, 18
overhead, 133
OWL, 33
OWL data properties, 33
OWL object properties, 33

parallel processing, 130
parallel programming models, 142
privacy, 193
privacy preservation, 194, 195, 210,
    211
Probabilistic Latent Semantic Analy-
    sis, 123

QoS-aware routing, 73

reduce function, 146
regression model, 116
Role-Based Access Control (RBAC),
    204

scalability, 132

security, 192
security best practices, 206
security breach, 199
self-speedup, 131
semantic interoperability, 17, 32
shared address space model, 142, 143
shared memory multiprocessor, 135
single system image, 138
social network, 79
speedup, 131
stationary time series, 118
super column family, 187
support, 112
syntactic interoperability, 17

task pallelism, 143
telehealth, 8
term frequency, 122
text mining, 120
thermal-aware routing, 73
time series, 115
time series: applications, 120
topic modeling, 123

UMA, 136
uniform memory access, 136

Vs of Big Data, 13, 44

WBAN, 51, 66
WBAN interference, 74
WBAN MAC layer, 72
WBAN network layer, 73
WBAN physical layer, 71
WBAN routing, 73
WBAN sensor, 70
wide-column stores, 168
WiFi, 71
work-optimality, 132

ZigBee, 71